General Preface to the Series

Because it is no longer possible for one textbook to cover the whole field of biology while remaining sufficiently up to date, the Institute of Biology has sponsored this series so that teachers and students can learn about significant developments. The enthusiastic acceptance of 'Studies in Biology' shows that the books are providing authoritative views of biological topics.

The features of the series include the attention given to methods, the selected list of books for further reading and, wherever possible, suggestions for practical work.

Readers' comments will be welcomed by the Education Officer of the Institute.

1979   Institute of Biology
                                                         41 Queen's Gate
                                                         London SW7 5HU

Preface

Man and other mammals living at sea level enjoy the benefits of a considerable head of pressure of oxygen driving it from the atmosphere to the mitochondria. When they ascend mountains, they become subjected to a lower barometric pressure and are deprived of an adequate supply of the gas. Lowlanders and the native Quechua highlanders of the Andes must undergo a remarkable series of changes in many systems of the body to adjust themselves to the new conditions, by the process of *acclimatization*. Indigenous high-altitude animals and perhaps the Sherpa highlanders of the Himalayas show characteristics of *adaptation* to the same environment. This book gives an account of the striking biological changes which are to be found in those who live in high places. It is based on a summary of the extensive world literature on high-altitude medicine and physiology available in specialist journals. This basis is tempered by the personal experience of the authors derived from four expeditions to the Peruvian Andes during the last decade. We should like to take this opportunity of thanking our many Peruvian friends in Lima and Cerro de Pasco for their great cooperation and kindness. We also wish to thank Denise Green and Robert Biggar for their help in the preparation of the manuscript.

Liverpool, 1979   D.H.
                                                         D.R.W.

Contents

The Institute of Biology's
Studies in Biology no. 112

Life at
High Altitude

Donald Heath

M.D., Ph.D., F.R.C.P., F.R.C.Path.
George Holt Professor of Pathology, University of Liverpool.
Honorary Professor of Pathology, Cayetano Heredia Medical School, Lima, Peru

David Reid Williams

L.R.P.S.
Department of Pathology, University of Liverpool

Edward Arnold

First published 1979
by Edward Arnold (Publishers) Limited
41 Bedford Square, London WC1B 3DQ

Paper edition ISBN: 0 7131 2754 6

Heath, Donald
    Life at high altitude.—(Institute of Biology. Studies in
    biology; no. 112 ISSN 0537-9024).
    1. Altitude, Influence of
    2. Man—Influence of environment
    I. Title   II. Williams, David Reid   III. Series
    612'.01441'5   QP82.2.A4

    ISBN 0-7131-2754-6

To Gareth

Printed in Great Britain by
Thomson Litho Ltd, East Kilbride, Scotland

1 The Physical Environment

The term 'high altitude' has no precise definition. This is illustrated very well by the fact that the elevations of 'high altitude research stations' throughout the world range from Jujuy in Argentina at 1260 m to Morococha in Peru at 4540 m. In this account 'high altitude' is taken to mean an elevation of 3000 m or more, because it is at this height that the majority of subjects ascending high mountains develop unequivocal signs and symptoms associated with the ascent. Mountainous areas approaching or exceeding 3000 m are to be found in many parts of the world (Fig. 1-1). Some of these areas are

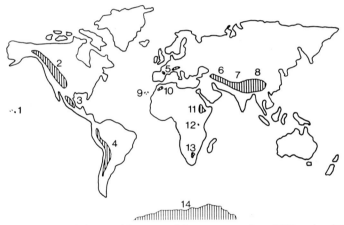

Fig. 1-1 Areas of the world approaching or exceeding 3000 m in altitude 1, volcanoes of Mauna Kea and Mauna Loa on Hawaii. 2, Rocky Mountains. 3, Sierra Madre. 4, Andes. 5, Pyrenees and Alps. 6, mountain ranges of Eastern Turkey, Iran, Afghanistan and Pakistan. 7, Himalayas. 8, Tibetan Plateau and Southern China. 9, volcano of Mount Teide on Tenerife in the Canary Islands. 10, Atlas Mountains. 11, high plains of Ethiopia. 12, Kilimanjaro. 13, Lesotho. 14, mountains of Antarctica.

populated, especially in the Andes and the Himalayas, and the people living there are exposed to physical factors not operative at sea level. Considered below are factors influencing life at high altitude.

1.1 Hypoxia

The percentage of O_2 in the atmosphere is the same at high altitude as it is at sea level. Indeed this percentage of 20.93% remains constant in the atmosphere up to an altitude of 110 000 m. However, since gas is compressible, the number of molecules a unit volume contains at sea level is greater than at high altitude, i.e. the barometric pressure decreases with increasing altitude. It follows that the partial pressure of oxygen in the atmosphere (PO_2—see p. 6) is progressively reduced with increasing altitude. At sea level the barometric pressure is 760 mm Hg and so PO_2 is 20.93% of that value, namely 159 mm Hg. There is a precise relationship between altitude, barometric pressure, and air (and hence O_2) pressure (Fig. 1-2). Shortage of O_2 is by far the most important adverse feature of the physical environment at high altitude for living organisms. The study of the physiology of man and mammals at high altitude is largely the study of their adjustment to a chronic deprivation of O_2. In common medical and physiological parlance, shortage of O_2 is termed 'hypoxia'.

1.2 Cold

Another environmental hazard to life in mountains is cold. Temperature falls with increasing altitude by about 1°C for every 150 m and this is independent of latitude. Latitude does influence the temperature of mountainous areas, for in tropical regions there is little seasonal change but much diurnal variation in temperature. The reverse is true of areas of higher latitude. In the Andes there is a striking difference in temperature in shadow and in direct sunlight. Ernst Schmidt climbed Everest in 1956 and removed his down-filled clothing at 8530 m because of the heat in the sunshine with low wind velocity.

1.3 Humidity

High mountain regions usually have a low temperature and low relative humidity, a combination which can prove very unpleasant to man. The profuse sweating may lead to dehydration and play some part in initiating thrombosis in the peripheral veins of high-altitude climbers. *Thrombosis* is the formation of a solid body from the elements of the flowing blood and consists of the deposition of blood platelets onto the lining of a blood vessel with the formation of a clot of fibrin in which the blood cells are trapped.

1.4 Solar radiation

There is increased exposure to solar radiation at high altitude. The clear mountain air permits the easy passage of such radiation to the earth's surface. The degree of solar heat absorption depends on the darkness of the clothing, fur or feathers, and the position of the individual. Snow increases the solar radiation by reflecting it. This

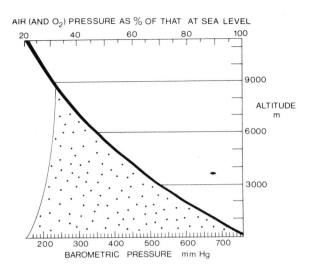

Fig. 1-2 The relationship between altitude, barometric pressure and air (and O_2) pressure as a percentage of that at sea level. (After FRISANCHO, A. R. (1975). Functional adaptation to high-altitude hypoxia. *Science*, **187**, 313.)

measure of a surface to reflect light is termed the *albedo*. It is less than 25% without snow but increases to 75 to 90% of the total solar radiation in its presence. The cornea may be damaged by excessive ultraviolet (UV) radiation reflected from the snow. This keratitis is known as *snow blindness* and may progress to blisters on the cornea. The subject becomes in effect 'blind' only in the sense that the intense pain and photophobia cause him to keep his eyes shut.

Whether mountain ranges are covered in snow or not depends on their geographical situation. Areas such as the western slopes of the Andes are desert-like due to the effect of the Humboldt water current in the Pacific. Others, like the eastern Himalayan range of Nepal, are subjected to heavy snow fall due to the combined effects of high altitude and the monsoon.

1.5 Ultraviolet radiation

This segment of solar radiation extends from 200 to 400 nm. At an altitude of 4000 m, UV radiation of wavelength 300 nm is increased by a factor of 2.5. The major determinant of the level of UV radiation received by an area is, however, the amount of sunlight it gets. Thus, sunny areas at sea level may receive more UV radiation than high-altitude regions.

1.6 Ionizing radiation

Man and animal species are subjected to natural ionizing radiation which may be cosmic or may arise from their terrestrial environment. At high altitude there is an increase in the levels of cosmic radiation which consists of extremely penetrating rays from outer space. High energy protons (positively-charged particles derived from the atomic nucleus) enter the earth's atmosphere to produce π mesons. These are heavy sub-atomic particles which decay to form μ mesons most of which survive down to ground level to form hard, penetrating radiation. Heavier K mesons and sub-atomic particles called hyperons are also involved. There is no evidence to suggest that increased cosmic radiation at high altitude brings about serious deleterious effects such as genetic damage.

1.7 Geographical situation and mountain zones

The environmental hazards referred to above will always be encountered on mountains at high altitude. Other hazards, however, will only be present if the geographical situation of the mountain range is appropriate. This applies especially to climatic factors such as the level of precipitation. Thus the western slopes of the Andes and the Karakorums are desert, while the Himalayas of Nepal are covered in ice and snow. The physical features of the environment in most mountainous areas change with increasing altitude so that well-defined zones can be recognized, each associated with a characteristic fauna and flora. In the Himalayas there are five zones: rain, forest, temperate, the Tibetan plateau and, at the highest altitude, what has been termed an 'Ice-Kingdom' of glaciers, crevasses, winds of hurricane force and temperatures as low as $-40\,°C$.

An important aspect of mountain regions is the accessibility of their higher reaches to man and mammals. In Peru, tourists, lowlanders and highlanders returning to their mountain home may reach altitudes exceeding 4000 m in very few hours by car or bus. There is then the risk of their developing acute mountain sickness or high-altitude pulmonary oedema (see §4.2). In contrast to this, the Himalayan peaks are inaccessible and high-altitude climbers are fully acclimatized before embarking on the conquest of their chosen mountain.

2 Transport of Oxygen from Air to Tissues

At rest, the tissues of the body consume some 220 to 260 ml of O_2 per minute. This figure is expressed at standard temperature and pressure and with the gas dry (i.e. STPD); by convention these conditions are taken to be $0°C$, 760 mm Hg, dry. There is an inexhaustible reservoir of the gas in the atmosphere, and the problem of providing an adequate supply of O_2 to the mitochondria where it will be used, lies in the complex nature of the route in the body along which the O_2 must travel to reach the cells. Thus, the process of respiration is a complex combination of four transport mechanisms. In *ventilation*, air flows through the trachea and bronchial tree to the alveolar spaces of the lung. In *pulmonary diffusion*, the air passes from the alveoli, through the alveolar capillary walls of the lung tissues, to reach the blood. O_2 is then carried by *blood transport* from the capillaries of the lung to those of the tissues. Finally, in the fourth stage – *tissue diffusion* – O_2 passes from the systemic capillaries to the intracellular mitochondria where it will be used. In healthy man at sea level this complex transport of the gas from atmosphere to mitochondria functions efficiently because of the great head of pressure which exists between the two: the PO_2 in the atmosphere at sea level is 159 mm Hg whereas the critical PO_2 for oxidative enzyme reactions in mitochondria is of the order of 1 to 2 mm Hg.

2.1 Oxygen gradients

At each of the four stages of respiration there is a fall in O_2 tension and the magnitude of these changes at sea level is shown in Fig. 2-1. The succeeding falls in the partial pressure of the gas at each stage are termed the 'O_2 cascade'. At high altitude the barometric pressure is diminished and hence with it the pressure difference of O_2 available for transport to the mitochondria. Theoretically, there are two mechanisms by which this shortfall in PO_2 in the atmosphere could be compensated. Tissue metabolism could be altered so that the biochemical demands for O_2 were less or, alternatively, the transport for the gas could be modified so that PO_2 was maintained at higher levels than would be anticipated. This modification of O_2 gradients so that the cascade is much less steep, is in fact the manner in which the human body becomes *acclimatized* to high altitude. It is not, however, the manner in which animals indigenous to mountain areas are *adapted* to the hypoxia of high altitude (see §2.6.5).

6 §2.2

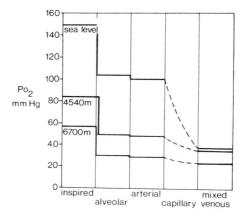

Fig. 2-1 Mean O_2 pressure gradients from inspired air to mixed venous blood in i) subjects native to sea level, ii) subjects native to 4540 m, and iii) climbers at 6700 m. This 'O_2 cascade' in subjects at high altitude is seen to be much less steep than in sea-level residents. Thus, although PO_2 in the atmosphere at high altitude is much less than at sea level, the final PO_2 achieved in the mixed venous blood of subjects at high altitude is not greatly diminished. (Based on data from HURTADO, A. (1964). Some physiologic and clinical aspects of life at high altitudes. In: *Aging of the Lung*, p. 257. Edited by L. Cander and J. H. Moyer. Grune and Stratton, New York, and from LUFT, U. C. (1972). Principles of adaptations to altitude. In: *Physiological Adaptations. Desert and Mountain*. Edited by M. K. Yousef, S. M. Horvath and R. W. Bullard. Academic Press, New York and London.)

In describing the transport of gases in the body it is necessary to use a system of physiological symbols. A series of primary symbols, denoting general physical quantities such as pressure, are represented by a large capital letter. Thus, pressure is represented as P. Secondary symbols are placed immediately after the primary ones and consist of small capital letters for localization in the gas phase. Thus PA = pressure of gas in the alveolar spaces of the lung. Lower case letters are used for localization in the blood phase. Thus Pa = pressure of gas in arterial blood. The chemical symbol for the gas in question is written as a subscript. Thus Pa_{O_2} = pressure of oxygen in arterial blood. When the chemical symbol qualifies a primary symbol alone, it follows immediately after the primary one. Thus PO_2 = pressure of oxygen. These symbols will be used throughout this account.

2.2 Hyperventilation

When air is breathed into the bronchial tree, it becomes humidified and saturated with water vapour which exerts a partial pressure of

47 mm Hg. Hence the PO_2 in *inspired* air at sea level is 20.93% of 760
-47 mm Hg, i.e. 149 mm Hg. This already represents a diminution of
10 mm Hg from the PO_2 in the atmosphere (20.93% of 760 mm Hg),
i.e. 159 mm Hg. Once in the alveolar spaces, O_2 diffuses through the
alveolar walls to the pulmonary capillaries while CO_2 diffuses out
from them into the alveolar spaces. As a result PO_2 in the alveolar
spaces is about 100 mm Hg and already a third of the O_2 gradient
transporting the gas to the mitochondria has been lost.

At each breath only some 15% of the alveolar air is replaced by
fresh air. At high altitude there is deeper breathing (*hyperventilation*)
and this elevates PA_{O_2}. Native highlanders, such as the Quechua
Indians of the Peruvian Andes, hyperventilate 25 to 35% above the
value for sea-level man. Newcomers to high altitude hyperventilate
within a few hours of ascent and this increases rapidly during the first
week at high altitude, the ventilation exceeding that of native
highlanders by 20%. Such deep breathing maintains an adequate O_2
tension in the alveolar spaces in the face of a low pressure of the gas in
the atmosphere. This increased depth in breathing is effected by a
greater tidal volume, i.e. each individual breath is deeper. An increase
in the *rate* of breathing does not occur until the newcomer ascends to
an extreme altitude of 6000 m. When the respiratory rate increases at a
lower altitude of 3000 to 4000 m, it has a more serious significance,
suggesting the early onset of acute mountain sickness.

The initial hyperventilation is due to stimulation of the peripheral
chemoreceptors such as the carotid bodies. Initially the degree of lack
of O_2 in the blood – *hypoxaemia* – which is necessary to stimulate
hyperventilation, is considerable. However, once acclimatization has
occurred increased breathing is stimulated by Pa_{O_2} as high as
90 mm Hg. This striking sensitivity of chemoreceptors remains forever.
In contrast, the chemoreceptors are insensitive to conditions of O_2
lack in highlanders born and living at high altitude.

2.2.1 Respiratory alkalosis

The increased depth of breathing washes out CO_2 and tends to lead
to a rise in blood pH. This condition, *respiratory alkalosis*, is corrected
by the renal excretion of excess bicarbonate restoring blood hydrogen
ion concentration, $[H^+]$, towards normal. After this slow com-
pensatory process has occurred, the subject is left with a Pa_{CO_2} that is
lower than normal, and a reduced blood bicarbonate concentration. It
has been suggested that the cerebrospinal fluid reacts far more rapidly
to acute exposure to hypoxia by not sharing in the general alkalosis. It
has been thought that it remains relatively acid due to active transport
of bicarbonate ions out of the cerebrospinal fluid through the choroid
plexus (the specialized tissue in the brain which forms the fluid). In
this way, the medullary CO_2 or $[H^+]$ receptors remain stimulated and

do not counteract the initial stimulation of ventilation by the carotid bodies as they would appear to do if sharing in the general respiratory alkalosis. However, this concept of such a homeostatic mechanism in the cerebrospinal fluid to control respiration has been widely challenged by various investigators who claim to have demonstrated a rise in the pH of the cerebrospinal fluid on acute exposure to high altitude.

2.2.2 Sustained hyperventilation: influence of CO_2

At sea level, ventilation is largely controlled by the level of CO_2. The response of ventilation to this gas is influenced by the prevailing PO_2, so that with increasing hypoxia the response curve of ventilation to CO_2 steepens. Hence, by using various levels of hypoxia, a 'fan of curves' may be produced (Fig. 2-2). On ascent to high altitude the fan of curves moves to the left so that, at an extreme altitude of 5800 m, its origin moves from 38 to 23 mm Hg, i.e. the respiratory centre responds at high altitude to a level of CO_2 reduced by almost half. Furthermore, it responds more briskly to any increment in CO_2. A fall in PO_2 still increases the response to CO_2. Hence, in highlanders the sensitivity to CO_2 remains high but that to hypoxia is blunted. Some authorities believe that a heightened sensitivity to CO_2 is an important factor in sustaining hyperventilation. The respiratory sensitivity to this gas increases in less than a day at high altitude and then continues to increase to the eighth day.

Carbon dioxide transport is modified in those living at high altitude: there is a fall in Pa_{CO_2} so that at 4540 m it is 33.0 mm Hg, in contrast to 40.1 mm Hg at sea level. This fall is, as noted above, compensated for by a proportional decrease in bicarbonate, so that blood pH is maintained within normal limits. The increased fraction of red cells (erythrocytes) in the blood at high altitude also modifies CO_2 transport: it leads to a greater participation of these cells in the process so that they carry increased levels of an unstable combination of CO_2 with an uncharged amino group of haemoglobin called carbamino-haemoglobin.

2.2.3 Influences on the control of breathing arising from higher centres in the brain

There is some evidence that the chronic hypoxia of high altitude modifies a central mechanism influencing the respiratory centres in the primitive brain-stem. It is thought that there is an inhibitory influence which arises from higher centres in the grey matter of the cerebral hemispheres and which can be removed to release an underlying facilitatory influence originating in the diencephalon. Early in acclimatization there may be arousal by the reticular formation, a

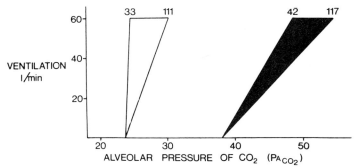

Fig. 2-2 The ventilatory response of a subject at sea level (filled triangle) and at 5800 m (open triangle) to the two levels of pressure of CO_2 in the alveolar space of the lung at the two altitudes. For each level of PA_{CO_2} the ventilatory response is shown for two levels of PO_2 which are indicated by numbers at the upper ends of the lines. At high altitude the respiratory centre responds to a level of CO_2 reduced to almost half of sea-level values. Furthermore, the response is brisker to any increment in CO_2. (From data of MILLEDGE, J. S. (1975). Physiological effects of hypoxia. In: *Mountain Medicine and Physiology*, p. 73. Edited by C. Clarke, M. Ward and E. Williams. Alpine Club, London.)

zone of nervous tissue which controls wakefulness, which accounts for hyper-responsiveness leading to symptoms of insomnia and irritability. The cortical influence develops more slowly to override the diencephalic facilitatory influence and the blunted hypoxic drive becomes apparent.

2.3 Pulmonary diffusion

When O_2 passes from the alveolar spaces to the blood in the pulmonary capillaries, it has to traverse the cells lining the alveolar spaces of the lung (i.e. the membranous and granular pneumocytes), the fused basement membrane of the alveolar-capillary wall, and the endothelial cells of the pulmonary capillaries (Fig. 2-3). Normally there is a drop in PO_2 in the blood of the pulmonary capillaries compared to that in the alveolar spaces. Employing the physiological symbols referred to earlier, this is termed the 'A-a difference' and at sea level it is between 5 and 10 mm Hg. In native highlanders this fall in PO_2 is lower and of the order of 2 mm Hg. This is, therefore, a further feature of respiratory acclimatization to high altitude facilitating diffusion of O_2 into the blood and diminishing the steepness of the O_2 cascade.

An increased internal surface area of the lung might be a factor in increasing pulmonary diffusing capacity and reducing the A-a difference. The high-altitude Quechua and Aymara peoples of the

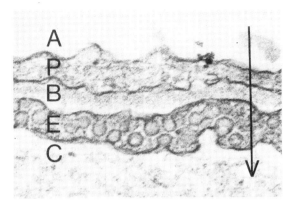

Fig. 2-3 Electron micrograph of the alveolar-capillary wall of the rat showing the ultrastructural components of the anatomical barrier to the diffusion of O_2 from the alveolar spaces of the lung into the blood. The direction of the O_2 diffusion is shown by the arrow. A, alveolar space. P, membranous pneumocyte. B, fused basement membrane. E, endothelial cell of pulmonary capillary. C, lumen of pulmonary capillary. (x 56 250).

Andes have a full chest and an increase in the volume of some compartments of the lung. This applies to the volume of gas remaining in the lung at the end of a normal expiration (functional residual capacity) and that remaining after a forced expiration (residual volume). Unfortunately, up to the present there are no quantitative microscopic studies of the internal surface area of the lung. The moderate elevation of pulmonary arterial pressure (described in §3.2) may also improve pulmonary capacity at high altitude.

2.4 Alveolar surface tension

There is one report of an increase in surface tension of lung extracts of mice after their acute exposure to a simulated altitude of 4270 m. However, the technique employed in this work has been challenged on the grounds that it releases a great deal of the fats from cells. The lipids released in such quantity may swamp the fatty compounds which lower surface tension because these specialized substances account for only 5 to 10% of the total lipids in the lung. It is of interest, however, that in the llama, (*Lama glama*), there is pronounced activity of the non-ciliated, so-called Clara cells of the respiratory bronchioles. These cells have been considered by some to be a secondary source of the lung surfactant, dipalmitoyl lecithin, which lowers surface tension in the alveolar spaces of the lung. Such cellular activity could be held to produce a sustained secretion of surfactant necessary to overcome a possible increased surface tension of high altitude.

Recent studies suggest that adjustments to respiratory physiology at high altitude are acquired and determined by environmental rather than genetic factors. Normal hypoxic ventilatory drive is developed in the native highlander up to the age of eight years before it is substantially lost during adult life. The 'vital capacity' (i.e. the greatest possible inspiration followed by the expiration of all the air within the lungs that is voluntarily possible) of the highlander outpaces that of sea-level children after the age of nine years.

2.5 Transport of oxygen to the tissues by the blood

The supply of O_2 to the tissues is a product of the cardiac output, the haemoglobin concentration, and the percentage O_2 saturation of systemic arterial blood. Requirements of O_2 may increase tenfold on exercise and these can be met, to some extent, by the heart pumping more blood per minute around the body. However, at high altitude the quantity of O_2 transported to the tissues is considerably enhanced by elevation of the haemoglobin concentration of the blood.

In the native Quechua highlanders of the Andes the *haemoglobin concentration* rises from sea-level values of around $15 \, g \, dl^{-1}$ to some $20 \, g \, dl^{-1}$. The *red cell count* rises from 5.1 to $6.4 \times 10^{12} \, l^{-1}$. The percentage of the blood volume formed by red cells, the *haematocrit*, rises from 45 to 60%. The *reticulocyte count* rises from 18 to 45 $\times 10^9 \, l^{-1}$: this counts the number of young red cells in the blood which still contain a network (or reticulum) of threads of the basophilic ribonucleic acid. The increase of these young red cells at high altitude indicates the stimulating effect of the hypoxic environment on the bone marrow. There is considerable variation in the haemoglobin levels of native Andean highlanders. The bone marrow shows hyperplasia of the precursors of the red cells. In contrast, the precursors of the white cells, and the blood-platelet-producing cells, the megakaryocytes, remain normal in number and maturation. In lowlanders during the first one or two weeks at high altitude, there is an initial decrease of 15 to 20% in plasma volume which results in an increase in circulating haemoglobin. The high haemoglobin level is maintained by a daily red cell production some 30% higher than that of lowlanders at sea level. The remarkable sensitivity of the regulatory mechanisms which control blood-forming (erythropoietic) activity is demonstrated by the fact that within two hours of exposure to high altitude red cell production increases. The iron turnover rate, in mg per day per kg body weight, increased from 0.37 to 0.54 in one group of lowlanders taken to 4540 m. In one or two weeks this rate rises to 0.91, so that erythropoietic activity is about three times higher than at sea level. Thereafter the rate falls, but it is still elevated after six months. Even after a year's residence at high altitude the erythropoietic balance is still not achieved, and this makes it clear that the rise in haemoglobin level is one of the slower components of acclimatization. The degree of red cell formation is related to the level of altitude. Up to an elevation of 3660 m the haemoglobin level increases in a linear relation to altitude. There is, however, a limit. Under conditions of extreme hypoxia, such as occurs at around 5800 m, there begins a decrease in the formation of haemoglobin. There is a relation between haematocrit and the age of permanent residents at different altitudes. Thus, a haematocrit of 75% which is accompanied by symptoms of chronic mountain sickness (see §4.5), is predictable at an age of 30 years at Morococha (4540 m), but at 63 years at Cerro de Pasco (4330 m). Iron absorption increases three to four times during early exposure to high altitude and the maximum is reached after one week. Conversely, there is a decrease in iron absorption during descent from high altitude reaching a minimum of one fifth of normal in three weeks. Greatly elevated levels of haemoglobin should not be regarded as a feature of a special 'high-altitude man' for while they are high in the Quechuas of the Andes they are not in the Sherpas of the Himalayas. This may be related (see §6.6), to the possibility that whereas the Quechuas are *acclimatized*, the Sherpas are *adapted* to high altitude.

2.6 Oxygen release to the tissues

So far this account has been concerned with the *quantity* of O_2 carried by the increased concentration of haemoglobin at high altitude, but it is clear that an equally important property is its ability to release that O_2 to the tissues. Whereas an enhanced affinity of haemoglobin will enable more O_2 to be carried to the tissues, a decreased affinity will increase the yield of the gas there, maintaining an adequate PO_2 for transport to the mitochondria. Central to this problem is the *oxygen-haemoglobin dissociation* $(O_2 - Hb)$ *curve*, the sigmoid shape of which is a reflection of the molecular events concerned with the oxygenation of the haemoglobin molecule (Fig. 2-4). Crystallographic techniques show that oxyhaemoglobin has a slightly different configuration from that of deoxyhaemoglobin: in the former, the pair of alpha chains and the pair of beta chains are slightly closer together. The combination of an O_2 molecule with a haem group alters the position of the ferrous iron in the haem ring, changing in turn the position of certain amino acids and changing the affinity for O_2 in the haem group in the neighbouring subunit chain. Thus, the uptake of each O_2 molecule in turn enhances the uptake of more. The position of the (O_2-Hb) curve is given by the PO_2 in plasma associated with 50% O_2 saturation of blood, when half the

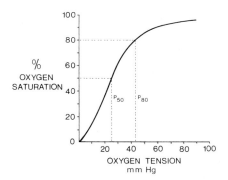

Fig. 2-4 The oxygen-haemoglobin dissociation (O_2–Hb) curve, relating the percentage of O_2 saturation of blood to the partial pressure of O_2 in the plasma. The position of the curve is given by the PO_2 associated with 50% O_2 saturation of blood. This is known as the P_{50}. The PO_2 associated with 80% O_2 saturation of blood is called the P_{80}. When the curve shifts to the right, the P_{50} rises, and when it shifts to the left, the P_{50} falls.

total haem groups are combined with O_2 at 37°C and pH 7.4. This is known as the P_{50} (Fig. 2-4).

2.6.1 Rightward shift of (O_2–Hb) curve in acclimatization

In native highlanders in the Andes, and in those who have acclimatized to high altitude, there is an increase in P_{50} and a shift of the (O_2 – Hb) curve to the right. This maintains a higher PO_2 and hence an adequate level of O_2 diffusion in the tissues. There is a higher value of PO_2 for every value of saturation and thereby a requisite PO_2 further along the capillary. Below an elevation of 3500 m this rightward shift of the curve offers a substantial advantage, but at higher altitudes the adequate release of O_2 to the tissues is more than counterbalanced by the inadequate affinity of haemoglobin for the gas and the inadequate uptake of O_2 in the lungs. Thus, at extreme altitude the most favourable response is a shift of the (O_2 – Hb) curve to the left.

2.6.2 2,3 diphosphoglycerate

Certain conditions stabilize the deoxy shape of the haemoglobin molecule favouring O_2 release. These include $[H^+]$ ions, CO_2, and 2, 3 diphosphoglycerate. 2, 3 DPG is generated by the anaerobic glycolytic pathway and each erythrocyte contains some 15μ moles per g of haemoglobin. It is able to enter the core of the haemoglobin molecule, when it is in the deoxy form, between the β chains, binding itself to each. This stabilization of the deoxy form favours O_2 release. Levels of 2, 3 DPG rise in people living at high altitudes causing the (O_2-Hb) curve to be shifted to the right. This is the hallmark of acclimatization in subjects living at altitudes of up to 5000 m. There is evidence to suggest that the altitude-induced increase in 2, 3 DPG is the result of alkalosis accompanying exposure. Experiments in rats show that the capacity for producing adequate and rapid rise in 2, 3 DPG concentration falls off with increasing age.

2.6.3 The increased Bohr effect

Quechua Indians show an increased *Bohr effect*, i.e. a greater decrease in affinity of haemoglobin for O_2 at the lower tissue pH. In one experiment the typical 'shift to the right' of the (O_2-Hb) curve was noted at pH 7.4 and pH 6.7. However, in the latter case the mean P_{50} and P_{80} values (the PO_2 required for 50% and 80% saturation of haemoglobin) of Europeans at high altitude are lower than those of native highlanders. Thus, in native highlanders of the Andes, the Bohr effect is increased at P_{50} and even more so at P_{80} (Fig. 2-5). There is

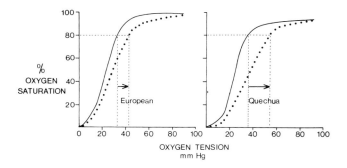

Fig. 2-5 Compared to Europeans the Quechua Indians show an increased Bohr effect, so that there is a greater decrease in affinity of haemoglobin for O_2 at the lower tissue pH of 6.7 (···) compared to a pH of 7.4 (–). Note the greater increase in the value for P_{80} with the fall in pH in the case of the Quechuas. This means that in the hypoxic conditions of life at high altitude there is a higher PO_2 available for use by the tissues where the pH is lower.

no modification of the haemoglobin molecule to explain this increased Bohr effect which aids acclimatization because it enhances the effect of the already rightward shift of the (O_2-Hb) curve in liberating an even higher level of PO_2 in the plasma at each level of O_2 saturation of blood. This will be apparent from study of Fig. 2-5.

2.6.4 Leftward shift of (O_2-Hb) curve at extreme altitude

At extreme altitudes exceeding 5800 m, the rightward shift of the (O_2-Hb) curve, associated with an increase of 2, 3 DPG within the red cell and an increased unloading of O_2 to the tissues, becomes unfavourable and eventually dangerous. This is because such a rightward shift exacerbates the dangerous degree of arterial un-saturation and introduces the possibility of severe hypoxaemia and death. At simulated extreme altitudes of 9180 m rats survive best if their drinking water is adulterated with 0.5% sodium cyanate which irreversibly changes the amino groups of haemoglobin to increase its affinity for O_2, thus shifting the (O_2-Hb) curve to the left. Such rats sustain a big decrease in 2, 3 DPG. Rats treated with carbon monoxide before exposure to extreme altitude and showing a fall in P_{50} but no change in 2, 3 DPG levels, have a lower survival rate than cyanate-treated animals but fare better than rats previously acclima-tized by exposure to chronic hypoxia with a shift of the (O_2-Hb) curve to the right.

2.6.5 Biological significance of shifts in the (O_2-Hb) curve

In summary, a *shift of the curve to the right* implies a lowered affinity of haemoglobin for O_2 with elevated levels of 2, 3 DPG. This means that O_2 unloading at the tissues is facilitated, maintaining an elevated PO_2 in association with some loss of O_2 saturation of the haemoglobin. This system is characteristic of *acclimatization* allowing survival at high altitude, but it is not so advantageous under conditions of extreme hypoxia. It is typical of the Quechuas who show natural acclimatization (Fig. 2-6).

On the other hand, a *shift of the curve to the left* implies increased affinity of haemoglobin for O_2, so that O_2 transport and haemoglobin saturation are enhanced at the expense of O_2 unloading at the tissues (Fig. 2-6). Such a system is found in indigenous high-altitude animals (see Chapter 5) and is characteristic of *adaptation* in contrast to acclimatization. It may also be induced artificially in laboratory animals (see § 2.6.4). A shift of the (O_2-Hb) curve to the left favours survival at extreme altitudes.

2.7 Tissue diffusion

The final area in which respiratory acclimatization to high altitude takes place is tissue diffusion. At sea level, there is a diffusing pressure of O_2 of some 30 mm Hg from the venous end of the capillary to the immediate vicinity of the mitochondria whose critical PO_2 is of the order of 1 to 3 mm Hg. At high altitude, there is some fall in the partial pressure of O_2 in the venous end of the capillaries. A fall of 10 to

16   § 2.7

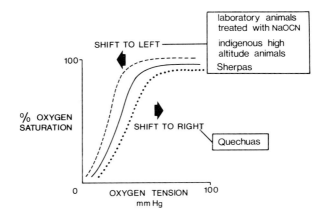

Fig. 2-6   Diagram to illustrate that in acclimatized Quechua Indians there is
a shift to the right of the (O_2–Hb) curve. However, in adapted indigenous
high-altitude animals the curve shifts to the left. A leftward shift has also been
reported in Sherpas and may be induced experimentally by treatment with
sodium cyanate (NaOCN).

15 mm Hg here would seriously endanger the survival of cells at the
periphery of the surrounding cylinder of tissue being provided with
O_2, unless further factors facilitating diffusion of O_2 to the
mitochondria operated.

2.7.1   Factors facilitating diffusion of oxygen

Increased capillary density. Capillary counts in acclimatized animals
have demonstrated an increased number of capillaries per unit of
tissue in the cerebral cortex, skeletal muscle and heart muscle
(myocardium). An added component of acclimatization demonstrated
in the skeletal muscle of dogs appears to be a significant decrease in
size of muscle fibres, thus again diminishing the distance over which
the O_2 has to diffuse to reach mitochondria (Fig. 2-7).
Amount of myoglobin in the tissues. Oxygen passes from the systemic
capillaries to the mitochondria by the very slow process of diffusion.
There is some evidence that the rate of diffusion is enhanced by the
increased amounts of tissue *myoglobin*. Myoglobin is a protein found
within cells; it has a molecular weight of about 17 500 and consists of
a single chain of 152 amino-acid residues and one iron-containing
haem group. It is of relevance to high-altitude studies because it has
the property of combining loosely and reversibly with O_2. Myoglobin
will combine with O_2 even when tissue PO_2 is very low. Thus when
PO_2 is 10 mm Hg, haemoglobin is only 10% saturated, whereas
myoglobin is 70% saturated. The generally accepted view, therefore, is

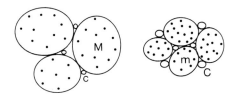

Fig. 2-7 Diagram illustrating some of the microanatomical changes in muscle which occur during acclimatization to high altitude. The situation at sea level is shown in the figure to the left, while that at high altitude is illustrated in the figure to the right. At high altitude the diameter of the muscle fibres decreases (M → m), while the blood capillaries supplying the fibres increase in size and number (c → C). Thus the distance over which O_2 has to diffuse is reduced.

that myoglobin acts as a reserve store of O_2 which is available during periods of activity. There are variants of myoglobin resulting from single amino-acid substitution. There is about 4.5 mg of myoglobin per g of human psoas (the muscle which extends from the sides of the lumbar spine to the thigh bone), and assuming this to be a representative skeletal muscle, this implies that 10 to 12% of the total body iron of man is myoglobin.

Myoglobin occurs in high concentration in muscles which carry out sustained or periodic heavy work such as mammalian myocardium. In chicken, the leg muscles which walk and scratch for food are red and contain much myoglobin, but the pectoral muscles which are intermittently used are white. On the other hand, the pectoral muscles of flying birds which are constantly used are red. The amount of myoglobin in muscle depends on how hard the muscle works. Its content in the muscle of rats, pigs and racehorses is increased by habitual exercise. It is important to note that while myoglobin combines reversibly with O_2 it gives up the gas slowly. An increased myoglobin content of skeletal muscle at high altitude has been reported in man, dogs, guinea pigs and rats.

An alternative function for this increased amount of myoglobin at high altitude is that it facilitates diffusion of O_2 rather than act as a reserve store. It appears that haemoglobin molecules must move to facilitate the diffusion of O_2; the haemoglobins of earthworms have a molecular weight of three million and do not facilitate the diffusion of O_2. Myoglobin has a much lower molecular weight and is capable of this function. It seems more likely that O_2 is passed from one myoglobin molecule to another by the rotation of the molecules rather than by their movement from one situation to another. Haemoglobin molecules are, in fact, closely packed in an orderly lattice not allowing their free movement. There is evidence that the intracellular diffusion of oxygen which is facilitated by myoglobin is about six times as great as that achieved in physical diffusion. When a high-altitude animal such as the alpaca is brought down to sea level, it shows a progressive diminution in the content of myoglobin in its skeletal muscles.

2.7.2 Mitochondria

These are the subcellular respiratory units that account for the bulk of O_2 consumed by the body. It is conceivable that an increase in number of mitochondria would increase the probability of an O_2 molecule finding an enzyme site in a shorter time and would thus have an apparent effect of increasing intracellular diffusion capacity. One study in which mitochondria were separated from specimens of heart muscle from cattle suggests that there was a 40% increase in number of mitochondria compared to hearts from sea-level cattle. The mitochondrial size remained the same. Studies on electron micrographs of myocardial mitochondria of rabbits and guinea pigs from Cerro de Pasco (4330 m) and sea level have, however, not confirmed the earlier work. Thus, quantitative electron microscopic analysis of tissue from the high-altitude animals showed no increase in mitochondrial volume expressed as a percentage of cytoplasmic volume. The number of mitochondria per ml of cytoplasm was not increased in the Peruvian animals and there was no significant increase in the surface area of outer and inner mitochondrial membrane expressed per ml of cytoplasm.

3 Effects of Sustained Hypoxia on the Body

3.1 Enlargement of the carotid bodies

It is now generally accepted that the carotid bodies and the smaller nodules of chemoreceptor tissue scattered throughout the body, such as the minute 'aortico-pulmonary bodies' in proximity to the aorta and pulmonary trunk, monitor the degree of O_2 saturation of systemic arterial blood. Since the major environmental hazard of life at high altitude is chronic hypoxia, one would anticipate that there would be disturbances of the form and function of the carotid bodies of mountain dwellers. In contrast to the situation at sea level, there is a definite progressive increment in the weight of the carotid bodies with age at high altitude (Fig. 3-1). Thus, the carotid bodies of the Quechua Indians of the Peruvian Andes are larger and heavier than those of mestizos living on the coast. The carotid bodies of guinea pigs, cattle, rabbits and dogs are significantly larger in the Andes. Experimental studies simulating high altitude in decompression chambers have shown that the enlargement of the carotid bodies of the rat exposed to hypoxia is rapidly reversible on return to sea-level conditions.

3.1.1 Histological changes

Chemoreceptor tissue is composed of two types of cell: (1) the *chief* or *type I*, cell, about 13 μm in diameter with a round nucleus 7 μm in diameter, and with palely eosinophilic cytoplasm and of ill-defined outline; (2) the *sustentacular* or *type II*, cell, an elongated supporting cell which may be related to Schwann cells of nerve sheaths. It is the chief cells which increase in number and contribute towards the enlargement of the carotid bodies in hypoxia. They show vacuolation of their cytoplasm. In cattle at high altitude the growth of chief cells is so pronounced that the appearances resemble the tumour of chemoreceptor tissue, the *chemodectoma*.

3.1.2 Chemodectoma

Amongst the human population of Peru chemodectomas are ten times more frequent at high altitude than at sea level. There is an association of such tumours with the papillary and follicular type of cancer of the thyroid in Mexico. Enlargement of the carotid bodies occurs in human patients with lung diseases such as chronic bronchitis and emphysema in which the alveolar sacs, or the

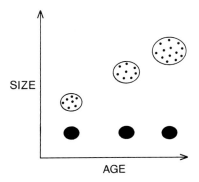

SIZE

AGE

Fig. 3-1 This diagram illustrates that the carotid bodies at sea level, indicated by solid ovals, are small and remain so throughout life. In contrast, the carotid bodies of the highlander, indicated by stippled ovals, are enlarged and increase in size with age.

respiratory bronchioles leading into them, become cystic and thus interfere with diffusion of O_2 to the pulmonary capillaries. As a result, such diseases lead to hypoxia similar to that experienced by highlanders. Detailed quantitative microscopic studies reveal that much of the enlargement of carotid bodies in animals exposed to acute hypoxia is due simply to congestion of blood vessels.

3.1.3 Ultrastructure

The chief cells of the carotid body contains neurosecretory vesicles. In sea-level subjects these vesicles have a dense solid central core which stains with osmium salts, and the cells are thus said to be osmiophilic. Around this osmiophilic core is a clear halo which has an outer limiting membrane. At high altitude small vacuoles are formed around the vesicles and the core in the centre of the vesicle shrinks and becomes paler and excentric so that the surrounding clear halo is broader and finally cystic. (Fig. 3-2.) In extreme hypoxia the vacuoles move to the edge of the cell and are discharged. The dense-cored vesicles may be concerned with chemoreception and, specifically, with monitoring of the O_2 content of the blood or, alternatively, with the secretion of a hormone. Thus the functional significance of these ultrastructural changes is at present obscure: it is not clear whether they represent the ultrastructural counter-part of a disturbance of a chemoreceptor or of an endocrine function.

3.1.4 Biogenic amines

The four amines isolated so far in the carotid bodies are dopamine (3, 4 dihydroxy-phenylethylamine), serotonin (5, 6 hydroxytrypta-

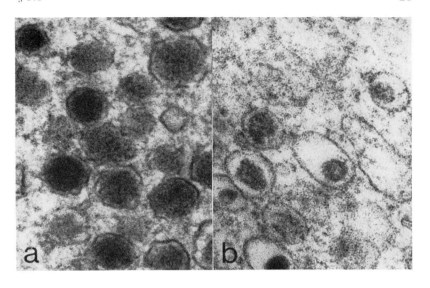

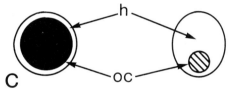

Fig. 3-2 Electron micrographs of the carotid body from: (**a**) a guinea pig born and spending all its life at sea level, and (**b**) a guinea pig born and living at an altitude of 4330 m. (Both micrographs × 75 000.) In the lowland guinea pig the neurosecretory vesicles are seen to consist of a dense osmiophilic core with a surrounding halo and a limiting outer membrane. In the high-altitude guinea pig, the inner cores of the vesicles are shrunken and the surrounding haloes enlarged so that the vesicles are transformed into vacuoles. These ultrastructural changes are associated with a loss of 'hypoxic drive' so that the native highlander becomes less responsive to O_2 deprivation than the lowlander. (**c**) Diagram to illustrate the ultrastructural changes in the neurosecretory vesicles of the carotid body on exposure to high altitude. The core of the vesicle at sea level is large and central and stains deeply with osmium salts; this osmiophilic core (oc) is surrounded by a narrow clear halo (h). At high altitude this core becomes smaller, paler and excentric and the narrow halo is transformed into a microvacuole.

mine), norepinephrine and epinephrine. Their percentage content in one study was found to be respectively 64, 18.8, 14.8 and 2.5. A similar unusually high concentration of dopamine is found only in parts of the brain such as the basal ganglia of the central hemispheres. In rats, those cells in the carotid bodies which contain small neurosecretory vesicles (47–55 nm) store norepinephrine, whereas those which contain large vesicles (63–78 nm) store dopamine. It has been postulated that secretion of dopamine from chief cells acts as an inhibitory transmitter. Under conditions of hypoxia, such as occur at high altitude, the release of dopamine from chief cells is thought to be reduced allowing nerve endings to return to their depolarized state. This depolarization may cause release of a neurotransmitter, perhaps acetylcholine, from the efferent synapses of the nerve terminals. This acts on chief cells reducing further still the rate of dopamine secretion. Hence hypoxaemia initiates a vicious circle of decreased dopamine secretion, increased depolarization and increased discharge frequency. This view has not gained universal acceptance.

3.1.5 Blunted ventilatory response to hypoxia

The enlargement of the carotid bodies which occurs at high altitude is associated with a blunted ventilatory response to hypoxia. Genetic factors are unlikely to be the basis for this. Two factors that do appear to be of importance are the age of the subject at the time of exposure to the hypoxia, and the duration of the exposure. When infants are exposed to hypoxia their chemoreceptors become insensitive to it. Reduction of the ventilatory response occurs during prolonged residence at high altitude, and appears to be irreversible. It is tempting to relate enlargement of the carotid bodies (with the associated histological and ultrastructural features described above) to the blunted ventilatory response. It seems likely that augmented carotid body size and weight with increasing age of highlanders is related to progressive insensitivity of these chemoreceptors.

3.2 Pulmonary hypertension

Exposure to the chronic hypoxia of high altitude brings about constriction of the vascular smooth muscle of the pulmonary circulation, but relaxation of the muscle of the systemic vasculature. Healthy man born and living at high altitude has some degree of raised blood pressure in the arteries of the lung – *pulmonary arterial hypertension*. The elevation of the mean pressure in the pulmonary arteries is mild, say 28 mm Hg, compared to the sea-level value of 12 mm Hg. In young children between the ages of one and five years, the degree of pulmonary hypertension is considerably greater. The effects of high altitude on the pressure and flow of blood in the lung are more pronounced on exercise. The pulmonary hypertension of highlanders can be reversed immediately with the administration of O_2 or, over a longer period of time, by removal of the subject to sea level.

3.2.1 Constriction of pulmonary arteries (vasoconstriction)

The basis for the pulmonary hypertension in man, and certain species of animals such as cattle, living at high altitude, is the sustained constriction of the terminal portions of the arterial tree of the lung. This contraction of the small pulmonary arteries becomes associated with muscularization and constriction of the pulmonary arterioles (Fig. 3-3) which, unlike the pulmonary arteries, are normally

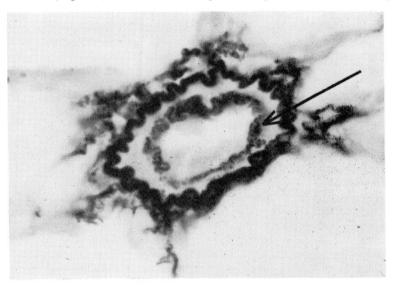

Fig. 3-3 Pulmonary arteriole from a rat exposed to a simulated high altitude. As in man, the normal arteriole has a wall consisting of a single elastic lamina. At high altitude these blood vessels develop a muscle coat (arrow) so that they come to resemble a systemic arteriole. This muscularization of pulmonary arterioles leads to the elevation of blood pressure in the lung which is so characteristic of men and cattle at high altitude. (Stained to demonstrate elastic tissue, × 750.)

devoid of muscle. It is interesting that the same muscularization of the distal portion of the pulmonary arterial tree is to be found in the foetus, not only of highlander-parents, but also of those at sea level. Physiologically, the foetus has much in common with the high-altitude dweller. Even at sea level the intrauterine umbilical arterial O_2 tension is about 20 mm Hg which corresponds to an atmospheric O_2 tension of 60 mm Hg which would be found at an elevation of about 7500 m.

The mechanism by which hypoxia affects the pulmonary vascular smooth muscle is controversial. For many years it has been accepted that alveolar hypoxia is a more potent vasoconstrictor than hypoxaemia (i.e. diminished arterial oxygen saturation of the blood). This being so, it has been thought that an agent lying between the alveolus and pulmonary arteriole was responsible for triggering off constriction of the blood vessels. For a long time the most likely candidate for such a rôle was the *mast cell*, a type of connective-tissue cell widespread in the body but with a tendency to accumulate around pulmonary blood vessels. The mast cell secretes various compounds some of which, like histamine, are capable of affecting the muscular tone of blood vessels. One school of thought has believed that histamine liberated from mast cells causes pulmonary arteries to constrict in states of hypoxia. This view is no longer so widely favoured, and a direct action of hypoxia on vascular smooth muscle is now thought likely. It is possible that the mechanism by which alveolar hypoxia could exert such an effect would need to involve some biochemical system of amplification since, in the lung, PO_2 far exceeds that required for the maintenance of function of mitochondria.

There is considerable individual variation in reactivity of the pulmonary circulation to hypoxia. Hyper-reactivity to hypoxia usually remains latent at sea level, but it may become manifest with increasing hypoxia. The muscularization of the pulmonary arterioles increases the resistance to the flow of blood through the lungs and hence increases the muscle mass of the right ventricle of the heart. Experimental studies on rats show that on relief from hypoxia such changes in the heart and blood vessels of the lung start to resolve in four to six weeks. In rats, age and sex have some influence on the effect of simulated altitude on the pulmonary vasculature. A greater tendency to muscularization of the pulmonary arterial tree is found in adult female rats.

3.2.2 Genetic factors

The susceptibility or resistance to the development of pulmonary hypertension at high altitude in cattle appears to be determined genetically (Fig. 3-4). Pulmonary arteriolar resistance increases to a much greater extent in the offspring of cattle known to be susceptible to the effects of high altitude. In man too, genetic factors appear to operate. Some highlanders show a degree of increased muscularization of their pulmonary arteries suggesting that they are unduly prone to develop pulmonary hypertension. The mildness of the elevation of pulmonary arterial pressure in the Quechua is probably a reflection of the fact that he has lived in the Andes for countless generations. On the other hand, there are communities like Leadville, Colorado (3100 m) which were settled barely a century ago. In such communities the population probably still contains families who are prone to develop pulmonary hypertension. Some children in this area have developed a fatal disease, characterized by severe pulmonary

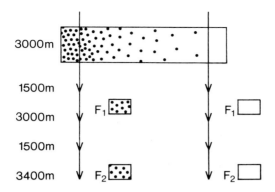

Fig. 3-4 Diagram to illustrate the genetic factor influencing the development of pulmonary hypertension in cattle at high altitude. The upper
rectangle illustrates the spectrum of reaction of the bovine pulmonary
vasculature to the hypoxia at 3000 m, the stippled end representing a strong
tendency to the development of a raised pulmonary arterial pressure, and the
clear end representing no tendency to pulmonary hypertension. Ten cattle
susceptible to pulmonary hypertension were taken to 1500 m. When their
offspring (F_1) were exposed to an altitude of 3000 m, they too showed
pulmonary hypertension. They were taken down to 1500 m and their offspring
(F_2) were taken to 3400 m where they too developed pulmonary hypertension.
In contrast, the offspring (F_1 and F_2 generations) of 15 cattle resistant to the
development of pulmonary hypertension, at no stage developed a raised
pulmonary arterial pressure.

hypertension and destructive changes in pulmonary arteries, called
primary pulmonary hypertension. It seems likely that they come from
such susceptible families. Functional closure of the patent ductus
arteriosus is hindered and delayed at birth at high altitude because of
the hypoxia.

3.2.3 Pulmonary trunk

The pulmonary hypertension of high altitude causes the pulmonary
trunk to remain thick-walled and muscular from birth. In experimental rats subjected to a simulated high altitude in a decompression
chamber, the individual smooth muscle cells in the process of
constriction show evaginations of their cytoplasm which are clear and
devoid of myofilaments and organelles (Fig. 3-5). At sea level, the
media of the pulmonary trunk is exposed to physiological pulmonary
hypertension during foetal life and, as a result, has an elastic tissue
pattern akin to that of the aorta (Fig. 3-6). During the first two years
of life at sea level this pattern becomes much less dense assuming an
open network which remains for the rest of life (Fig. 3-6). At high
altitude, due to the persistence of pulmonary hypertension throughout

life from birth, a 'persistent elastic tissue configuration' remains, so that the media of the pulmonary trunk has a histological appearance, chemical composition, and extensibility like that of the aorta (Fig. 3-6).

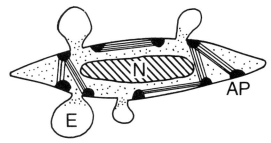

Fig. 3-5 Diagram of smooth muscle fibre showing the evaginations which project from its surface on constriction in response to stimuli such as the hypoxia of high altitude. The evaginations occur between attachment points (AP) for the actin filaments within the cytoplasm. When these filaments contract, the cytoplasm forms evaginations (E) which are devoid of organelles and myofilaments. The nucleus (N) is seen in the centre of the cell.

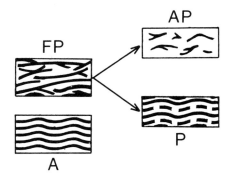

Fig. 3-6 Diagram to show the patterns of elastic tissue in the muscle coat (media) of the pulmonary trunk of the lowlander and of the highlander. In the foetus, the somewhat-branched elastic fibrils of the pulmonary trunk are tightly packed together (FP), and hence the pattern resembles that in the aorta (A) where the fibrils are long, unbranched and crowded together. The reason for this resemblance is that in the foetus the intravascular pressure is similar in the two arteries. After birth, the infant at sea level shows a considerable drop of blood pressure in the pulmonary trunk and as a result the elastic tissue becomes sparser and assumes the form of an open network of branched fibrils, the so-called adult pulmonary (AP) pattern. At high altitude this fall of pressure does not occur in the pulmonary trunk due to the constricting effect of the hypoxia of the atmosphere on the small arteries of the lung. As a result there remains a persistent pattern (P) of elastic tissue akin to that of the aorta.

3.3 Systemic circulation

The cardiovascular system influences the supply of O_2 to the tissues at high altitude by changes in the cardiac output and in the distribution of blood flow in the body. On ascent the heart rate increases excessively on exercise, but the stroke volume does not alter. As a result there is initially an increased resting cardiac output. After this time the rapid heart action remains but the stroke volume falls so that the cardiac output returns to normal. The diminished cardiac output characteristic of prolonged residence at high altitude is advantageous in the sense that the work load of the heart is not increased. However, this smaller systemic flow of blood is re-distributed so that vital organs and muscles are able to function effectively in the face of chronic hypoxia. Some tissues, such as the skin, have modest requirements of O_2 compared to organs like the heart, and at high altitude there is a redistribution of blood away from such areas to increase the O_2 reservoir for the remainder of the body. There is similarly a decreased flow to the kidneys at high altitude both in highlanders and in sojourners at elevation.

3.3.1 Blood volume

There is an increase in blood volume in those who live at high altitude, from about 80 to 100 ml per kg body weight. The increase in total blood volume is the result of increased red cell volume and the plasma volume is in fact lower in the highlander.

3.3.2 Systemic blood pressure

The arteries of the systemic circulation, which supplies every organ in the body except the lung, relax their tone on exposure to the chronic hypoxia of high altitude. As a result, the blood pressure in this circulation is lower in those living at high altitude than in sea-level residents. This is diametrically opposite to what takes place in the pulmonary circulation (see §3.2). Systemic hypertension, 'high blood pressure', is much commoner at sea level than at high altitude. When subjects move from the coast to mountainous areas their systemic blood pressure falls. Patients with high blood pressure at sea level improve on moving to high altitude.

3.3.3 Coronary circulation

After about ten days at high altitude, the newcomer from sea level experiences a diminution of the blood flow to the heart muscle through the coronary arteries by about a third. At the same time there is an increase in extraction of O_2 from coronary arterial blood by about 30% to maintain delivery of O_2 to the heart muscle. The coronary blood flow is also diminished in people living permanently at high altitude. Coronary artery disease and heart attacks resulting from it are both very uncommon. Native highlanders are 'low-risk subjects' because they are not subjected to mental stress so common in modern urban life. In addition, there is increased vascularization of the heart muscle in those living at elevation.

3.3.4 Electrocardiogram at high altitude

In those acutely exposed to the deprivation of O_2 of mountainous areas, studies of the electrical activity of the heart are consistent with increased strain on the right ventricle induced by the onset of pulmonary hypertension. In middle-aged lowlanders climbing at great heights, there is not uncommonly electrocardiographic evidence of temporary inadequate blood supply to the muscle of the left ventricle of the heart, this perhaps resulting from a combination of the hypoxia of the environment and slight inadequacy of the coronary arterial supply. Studies of the electrical activity of the heart muscle in native highlanders show a preponderance of the muscle of the right ventricle due to the sustained pulmonary hypertension of life at high altitude.

3.4 Endocrines

There is considerable disturbance of the endocrine organs during ascent to high altitude.

Adrenal cortex. Ascending to high altitude stimulates the adrenal cortex in a non-specific manner, with sharply increased secretion of its hormones, the 17-hydroxycorticosteroids, in the urine during the first week of exposure to mountain conditions. The precise nature of the stress is not known. The effect tends to be sustained for a considerable period and the resting level of corticosteroids in the plasma has been found to be elevated by some 60% even five weeks after return to sea level following a month's stay at high altitude.

Adrenal medulla. The activity of the adrenal medulla is also increased during early acclimatization. Urinary excretion of noradrenaline increases. Adrenal medullary activity in native highlanders is, however, normal.

Aldosterone. Increased levels of this hormone, secreted by the adrenal cortex, are known to be associated with a low sodium or high potassium diet and decreased extracellular volume. At high altitude there is an increased blood volume and this leads to stimulation of stretch receptors in the right atrium which depresses aldosterone secretion. The diminution in systemic blood pressure, already noted above, may in part be related to lowered secretion of this hormone.

Renin-angiotensin system. The renin-angiotensin system of hormones is concerned with the maintenance of blood pressure in the systemic circulation. Renin is secreted from the juxta-glomerular cells of the kidney and acts on the plasma protein, angiotensinogen, to produce the decapeptide angiotensin I. This is converted by an enzyme in the endothelial cells of the pulmonary capillaries to the octapeptide angiotensin II, which is a powerful vasoconstrictor capable of maintaining vascular resistance and pressure in the systemic circulation. There have been reports that this renin-angiotensin system is also involved in the development and maintenance of muscularization of the terminal portion of the pulmonary arterial tree in chronic hypoxia which is responsible for the pulmonary hypertension characteristic of life at high altitude. Blockade of angiotensin I conversion by SQ 20, 881, a synthetic nonapeptide, will significantly reduce in rats the extent of the increase in mass of the right ventricle and the muscularization of the pulmonary arterioles characteristic of the chronic alveolar hypoxia inherent in life at high altitude. Mice exposed to hypoxia develop increased granulation of the juxta-glomerular apparatus and elevated levels of angiotensin I—converting enzyme in lungs and serum during the second week of exposure. Interestingly, renin is formed in the same organ, and perhaps even the same cell, that synthesizes erythropoietin where the stimulus is known to be hypoxia.

Anterior pituitary. The continuous exposure of developing female rats to environmental hypoxia impairs the function of the anterior pituitary, retards body growth, and delays reproductive maturation.

Posterior pituitary. Increased flow of urine (*diuresis*) develops in persistent but mild hypoxia due to moderate altitude and appears to be due to diminution of circulating antidiuretic hormone from the posterior pituitary. This probably results from inhibitory impulses originating from receptors in the left atrium when it is distended by the increased blood volume resulting from acclimatization to high altitude. However, frequently on exposure to the severe hypoxia of high mountains there is a sudden discharge of antidiuretic hormone with the onset of *oliguria* (diminished output of urine) and acute mountain sickness.

Thyroid. This is one of the main regulators of O_2 consumption and so its function at high altitude is of considerable interest. Most studies have been carried out on animals and in conditions of acute hypoxia. Compared to sea-level controls, the thyroid glands of rats exposed to simulated high altitude show a statistically significant increase in the amount of colloid and a decrease in the amount of follicular epithelium. These histological changes are consistent with the reduced thyroid activity confirmed in a number of species. Both iodine retention in the whole animal and thyroid-concentrating power are decreased. This characteristic depression of thyroid function at high altitude may be of significance in acclimatization, increasing resistance of the myocardium to the effects of hypoxia.

Two factors complicate the study of the effect of high altitude on thyroid function under natural conditions. Firstly, mountain ranges are often *deficient in iodine* which leads to a lack of this element in the diet. This is a cause of enlargement of the thyroid gland and, as a result, goitrous swellings in the neck are a common sight in the peoples of the Himalayas and Karakorums. Such goitres can be prevented in highlanders by the injection of iodized oil which substantially corrects iodine deficiency for four to five years. The second complicating factor is the *coldness* of the mountain environment which itself affects thyroid function.

Insulin. Blood glucose levels are raised shortly after arrival at high altitude and persist for some months, but after two years they are significantly lower than at sea level. Native highlanders have reduced blood sugar and show increased glucose utilization. There is a reduction in the liver store of glycogen and an increased sensitivity to endogenous insulin at high altitude.

Testosterone. On exposure to high altitude the endocrine testis shows pronounced responses. There is an early fall in the urinary excretion of testosterone, the male sex hormone. The Leydig cells, which lie between the seminiferous tubules in the testes and are thought to be responsible for production of the male sex hormone, still maintain their normal response to an adequate stimulus.

3.5 Coagulation of the blood

There is a fall in the number of circulating blood platelets both in men ascending to mountainous regions and in animals exposed to simulated high altitude in a decompresseion chamber. In mice exposed to a simulated altitude of 5500 m, the platelet count falls to only 36% of control values by the end of twelve days. Such a fall appears to be due to either a decreased rate of production of thrombocytes or a structural or metabolic defect in platelets produced under conditions of hypoxia. Accumulation of platelets in the spleen has been shown not to be the cause of the diminution in the level of circulating blood platelets, termed thrombocytopenia. Decompression without hypoxia leads to a sharp fall in blood platelets. In one experiment, in which 16 men were decompressed to a simulated altitude of 6100 m, but were allowed to breathe O_2 with a PO_2 in the inspired air of 150 mm Hg, the platelet count fell by 10% and persisted for three days. In such decompression there is a reduction in platelet half-life with accumulation in the pulmonary vascular bed. No abnormality of the blood platelets at high altitude is revealed by electron microscopy.

The blood clots more readily at high altitude. Although there is a fall in the total number of blood platelets, there is an increase in the number of young, sticky platelets. There is a considerable shortening of the first stage of clotting. The increase in coagulability is countered by simultaneous increases in the level of proteolytic enzymes, called fibrinolysins, so that on moving to high altitude there is an abrupt fall in the plasma fibrinogen level due to its constant digestion. During continuous stay at high altitude the hypercoagulation state regresses.

3.6 Skin and nails

As part of the acclimatization to high altitude there is a redistribution of blood: it is shunted away from those areas where the extraction of O_2 is lower to other vital areas such as the heart and voluntary muscles where the O_2 extraction rate is high and a large supply of the gas is needed. The blood flow in the extremities is lower at high altitude than at sea level in both residents and newcomers. This appears to be the result of constriction of arterioles in the skin which thus increase the resistance to peripheral blood flow. At the same time, there is a constriction of the capacitance vessels of the skin, the veins and the capillaries, which diminishes the volume available for retention of blood in the skin.

The skin shows acute reaction to the increased UV radiation at high altitude, especially of wavelengths 380 nm and 300 nm. The acute effects result in a vivid reddening with vasodilatation which commonly proceeds to blistering and crusting. Subsequently, there is an increase in the number of cells in the epidermis called melanocytes which produce an excess of the black pigment melanin. Some of this pigment escapes into the dermis where it is engulfed by other cells called melanophores which accumulate there. In native highlanders who work chronically exposed to the UV radiation, thickening and furrowing of the skin complicate this pigmentation. Prolonged exposure leads to the deposition of thick interwoven fibres of a material called 'elastoid' in the dermis. There is also thickening of the horny layer of the skin, a process called *hyperkeratosis*, with the formation of plugs of keratin around hair follicles and sweat glands. The hyperkeratosis and increased density of melanin are probably a feature of acclimatization comprising barriers to the UV radiation. There is no convincing evidence that the excess of UV radiation brings about increased incidence of skin tumours – known as squamous and basal cell carcinomas and malignant melanomas. As already noted, the tumour of the carotid bodies, the chemodectoma, is commoner at high altitude, but this is due to an increase in the number of chief cells as a response to hypoxia, rather than to UV radiation. Small haemorrhages are to be found in the nails of healthy native highlanders and in those with chronic mountain sickness, and also in high-altitude climbers. They appear to be produced by a combination of hypoxia and minor injury.

3.7 Alimentary system and nutrition

Loss of body weight. Most newcomers to high altitude lose weight
because they lose their appetite (*anorexia*) due to nausea and
headache, and consequently eat less (*hypophagia*). On acute exposure
to altitude there is a distaste for fat, but an increased intake of
carbohydrate. The initial weight loss at high altitude is primarily due
to loss of stored body fat. Only on exposure to extreme altitude is
there wasting of muscle.

Urinary protein excretion. There is an increased excretion of protein in
the urine in native highlanders and in lowlanders undergoing
acclimatization to high altitude. The increase is small but unequivocal; it appears to be independent of glomerular filtration rate. At
birth, children at high altitude have renal glomeruli of normal size but
disproportionate enlargement occurs in childhood compared to sea-
level subjects. It is due to a proliferation of normal glomerular
elements.

Nutrient requirements at high altitude. When sea-level subjects ascend
mountains briefly for climbing, holidays, or temporary employment,
they eat less but the period of low intake of nutrients is so brief as not
to present a nutritional problem. So far as hydration is concerned,
with the onset of acute mountain sickness there is a diminished output
of urine and retention of water. On the other hand, at extreme
altitude, climbers become very dehydrated due to their high losses of
body water in the dry atmosphere. There is controversy as to the state
of hydration of the body once the initial period of acute exposure to
high altitude is over. Some observers say the body is *more* hydrated
and other say it is *less*. Analysis of carcasses of laboratory animals
exposed to simulated high altitude shows little or no change in body
water content. On acute exposure to the mountain environment there
is a net loss of sodium and a tendency to conserve potassium. This
leads to a reversal of the ratio of urinary sodium to potassium and
there is also a rise in the sodium/potassium ratio in saliva. These
changes in excretion of the two ions are probably related to the fall in
aldosterone secretion which occurs during the early stages of
exposure. Body stores of phosphorus are conserved like potassium on
exposure to high altitude.

Alimentary disease. During the Second World War it was noted that
some air crew personnel complained of dental pain when flying at
high altitudes. It is now generally accepted that such decompression
toothache occurs only when there is some pathological condition in a
vital pulp. At high altitude there is a tendency for small haemorrhages
to occur in the mouth and in the mucosal lining of the stomach where
they lead to an unusually high incidence of haemorrhage from the
stomach in such conditions as gastric ulceration. There is some
evidence that intestinal absorption is impaired in states of chronic

hypoxia, such as occurs on exposure to high altitude. There is, for example, a significant correlation between absorption of wood sugar (xylose) and the O_2 saturation of the blood. Haemorrhoids ('piles') are said to be unusually frequent in those undertaking high-altitude climbs. Any disease or medical procedure resulting in an air-filled cavity in the body is a hazard to those acutely exposed to high altitude. This is because, in accordance with Boyle's Law, pressure and volume vary inversely so that, as atmospheric pressure is reduced with altitude, any gas in the body cavities will expand. Even at a moderate altitude of 1830 m simulated in the cabin-pressure of modern aircraft, 100 ml of air will increase in volume to 130 ml. Such circumstances constitute a danger for patients with a disease of the lungs called emphysema which is often associated with large cysts on their lung surfaces. In the reduced cabin-pressure these cysts may rupture to allow air to escape into the chest cavity collapsing the lung. This condition is known as *spontaneous pneumothorax*.

3.8 Fertility and pregnancy

Demographic studies reveal a drift from the mountains during the present century. The Quechua and Aymara peoples of the Andes tend to be infertile and the basis for this is in part sociological and in part biological. Cohabitation between the sexes in the highlander occurs later and sexual relationships are less permanent than in mestizo low-landers. There are changes in the semen of men at high altitude: on ascent into mountainous areas there is a pronounced decrease in the number of sperms and an increase in non-motile and abnormal forms. Histological studies of the testes of animals subjected to severe simulated altitude reveal striking destruction of the germinal epithelium.

The onset of periods is delayed in school-age girls living at high altitude and there is increased incidence of menstrual disturbances, such as greater menstrual flow and painful and irregular periods. Even at sea level, the O_2 saturation in the umbilical arteries of the foetus is low, an expression of the resistance offered to the diffusion of O_2 by the tissue barrier of the placenta and to its own intrinsic O_2 utilization. At sea level, the umbilical arterial O_2 saturation is some 20 mm Hg, which corresponds to an atmospheric O_2 tension of about 60 mm Hg which would be found at an elevation of 7500 m. Thus, even at sea level the foetus can be regarded as a little highlander. At high altitude there is a distinct reduction in the O_2 tension in the capillaries of the uterus and in the maternal capillaries in the placenta. However, despite this, the O_2 tension in the umbilical vessels is similar to that reported for foetuses carried by ewes at sea level. It thus seems likely that the placenta of highlanders is modified in some way to decrease the resistance to the diffusion of O_2 across the placental barrier, or to increase the surface area across which gas exchange takes place. At high altitude, newborn children weigh less and placentas more, and the difference is most pronounced in female infants and in the offspring of women having their second or later pregnancies. In the highland woman having her first baby, the placenta is 23% heavier than in sea-level mestizos. The ratio of the weight of the placenta to that of the newborn infant is 0.144 on the coast at Lima but 0.192 at Rio Pallanga at high altitude in the Andes. An anatomical feature of the placenta is that it is subdivided into the areas called cotyledons. There are fewer of these in the placenta of the Quechua Indian woman delivering her baby at high altitude.

3.8.1 Foetal haemoglobin

Foetal haemoglobin (HbF) differs from the adult variety in that the polypeptide chains, usually termed β, are so different chemically that they are designated γ chains. It has a greater affinity for O_2 than the adult form, and its (O_2–Hb) curve is displaced to the left. Foetal and neonatal rats, mice, rabbits and puppies exposed to simulated altitude increase their production of HbF. Such species do not increase placental weight at high altitude. Other species, such as man, utilize the placental mechanism for adjustment to the hypoxia of high altitude.

3.8.2 Eggs and chicks at high altitude

Developing avian embryos lack the protection of a placenta. Decreased hatchability of chicken and turkey eggs at altitude above 1200 m has been recognized since the last century. Hypoxia leads to an increase in mortality rate throughout incubation but especially at an unusual time, namely during the second week of incubation. Embryonic growth in the chick is slowed by hypoxia. Differentiation is mainly affected between the tenth and thirteenth days, whereas growth is most involved after the sixteenth day, when half of embryonic growth normally takes place. Chicks prepare for their hypoxic environment at high altitude by an increased haematocrit at hatch.

4 Diseases of High Altitude

On exposure to high altitude the process of acclimatization begins and its physiological components give rise to unusual bodily sensations and symptoms. Thus, deeper breathing produces a feeling of breathlessness, and increased heart rate may give palpitations. These are the features of normal acclimatization, and they are reversed immediately by the inhalation of O_2. There are, however, more serious complications that can occur on exposure to high altitude.

4.1 Acute mountain sickness

A large proportion of those ascending into mountainous areas develop *acute mountain sickness*, also termed *soroche* in Peru and *puna* in Bolivia. It does not develop on immediate exposure to hypoxia, but follows a time lag of 6 to 96 hours. It is not due to deprivation of O_2 *per se*, but to a redistribution of body water that such hypoxia produces. It is commonly accepted that severe hypoxia leads to a decreased output of urine in many going to high altitude, this being the result of hypersecretion of anti-diuretic hormone (Fig. 4-1). The water retention is associated with shunting of blood away from the extremities with pooling in the lungs and brain leading to *oedema* (an excessive extravascular accumulation of fluid) of these organs, and there is also congestion of the splanchnic area (Fig. 4-1). This gives rise to symptoms related to these areas – nausea, vomiting, breathlessness and headache (Fig. 4-2). There may also be excessive secretion of the pituitary hormone, adrenocorticotrophic hormone (A.C.T.H.), which stimulates the adrenal glands to secrete more steroid hormones. The two sexes are equally affected. Incapacitating illness is likely to be short and measured in days rather than weeks, but the condition must not be regarded lightly for it may develop rapidly into high-altitude pulmonary or cerebral oedema. The newcomer to high altitude commonly experiences, as part of acute mountain sickness, feelings of fatigue and a desire to sleep which are quite disproportionate to the degree of physical activity he has undertaken. During sleep, breathing may become periodic (Cheyne-Stokes respiration). It is not established whether the orthodox or paradoxical (rapid eye movement, R.E.M.) type of sleep predominates in the early stages of acclimatization. The best way of avoiding acute mountain sickness is not to ascend too high too fast, and modern views as to what constitutes a safe rate of ascent are given in the next section. Sometimes the drug acetazolamide is given to produce a copious flow of urine and thus

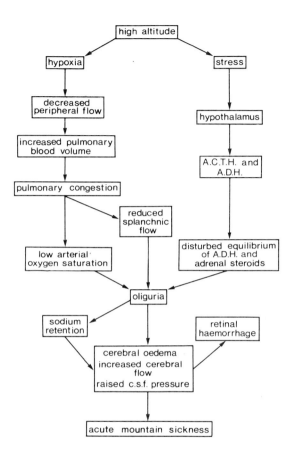

Fig. 4-1 Diagram to illustrate the factors that may be involved in the development of acute mountain sickness. It is based on the experience and hypothesis of I. Singh who had the opportunity to study may cases which occurred in the Himalayas in Indian soldiers during the border dispute with China. Hypoxia leads to increased pooling of body water in the lungs at the expense of blood supply to the periphery; it also gives rise to a diminished output of urine (oliguria). Stress leads to an increased secretion of antidiuretic hormone (A.D.H.) which also leads to oliguria. The oliguria and retention of sodium ions lead to waterlogging of the brain (cerebral oedema) as well as of the lung. This raises the pressure of the cerebrospinal fluid which leads to retinal haemorrhage as well as to the cerebral symptoms of acute mountain sickness. Stress also leads to an increased secretion of the pituitary hormone, adrenocorticotrophic hormone (A.C.T.H.), which causes the adrenal glands to secrete more steroid hormones. (See SINGH, I. *et al.* (1969). Acute mountain sickness. *New England Journal of Medicine*, **280**, 175.)

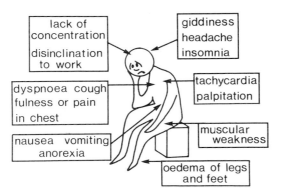

lack of
concentration
disinclination
to work

giddiness
headache
insomnia

dyspnoea cough
fulness or pain
in chest

tachycardia
palpitation

nausea vomiting
anorexia

muscular
weakness

oedema of legs
and feet

Fig. 4-2   The symptoms of acute mountain sickness. (Tachycardia – increased heart rate ; dyspnoea – breathlessness.)

avoid the retention of body water which is the basis of acute mountain sickness. This is what is called 'prophylactic treatment' but it has to be admitted that it is not so effective as ascending slowly.

4.2 High-altitude pulmonary oedema

Acute mountain sickness may develop into high-altitude pulmonary oedema in which the lungs become flooded with retained and redistributed body water. This produces intense breathlessness with the production of copious amounts of blood-stained watery froth at the mouth. It must be regarded as a medical emergency of the first order as it may lead rapidly to death. It is likely to occur in those engaging in too much physical activity too soon after arrival at high altitude. It is especially likely to occur in healthy young men and boys, and hence it is a hazard of skiing and climbing at high altitude. High-altitude pulmonary oedema is also especially likely to occur in those who have become acclimatized to hypoxia over a long period and who then descend to sea level only to return to high altitude again. The disease is a risk, therefore, for highlanders who return to their homes after a vacation at sea level. There are no racial differences in predisposition to the disease. When an X-ray of the chest is taken, the appearances are simply those of coarse shadowing predominantly at the roots of the lung, so that there is nothing special to differentiate this type of lung oedema radiologically from any other. In this disease, there is a raised blood pressure in the pulmonary arteries, but normal pressure in the pulmonary veins and left atrium. Electron microscopic studies of the lungs of rats subjected to simulated high altitude in decompression chambers, reveal small fluid-filled cysts which project into the lumens of the pulmonary capillaries. They appear to be formed by collection of fluid in the fused basement membranes of the

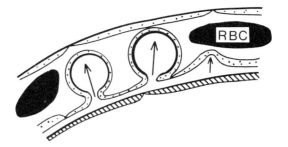

Fig. 4-3 Diagram to illustrate the mode of formation of fluid-filled cysts in the pulmonary capillaries in cases of simulated high-altitude pulmonary oedema in rats investigated in a decompression chamber. The cytoplasm of the endothelial cells of pulmonary capillaries is indicated by stipples. This cytoplasm is greatly distended over the cysts which form from oedema of the fused basement membrane of the alveolar capillary wall and project (arrows) into the capillaries containing red blood cells (RBC). The cytoplasm of the pneumocytes lining the alveolar spaces is indicated by cross-hatching. It is possible that fluid-filled cysts of this sort occur in human cases of high altitude pulmonary oedema.

alveolar wall, and they distend the cytoplasm of the endothelial cells of the pulmonary capillaries over them as they bulge inwards (Fig. 4-3). Sometimes, in individuals dying from this disease, agglutinations of blood platelets and fibrin and even small focal solidifications of blood (microthrombi) are found in the capillaries of the lung. It is far better to take steps to avoid this serious condition by not ascending too rapidly than to treat it once it has developed. Modern authorities tend to become progressively more conservative as to what constitutes a safe rate of ascent. A rate as low as 150 m a day above an altitude of 2750 m is now frequently advocated. Treatment of the established condition comprises, first and foremost, immediate descent to a much lower altitude, preferably sea level. Oxygen should be administered at a rate of 6–8 l min^{-1} while this descent is taking place. Powerful drugs designed to increase the flow of urine – diuretics, such as frusemide and bumetanide have been given to clear the oedema fluid but their use is controversial. If high altitude pulmonary oedema is not treated promptly and effectively, it may prove fatal.

4.3 Cerebral oedema

The worsening oedema of acute mountain sickness may involve the brain instead of, or as well as, the lungs. This leads to increasingly severe headache and perhaps to serious complications in the nervous system such as incoordination of muscle movement and speech, hallucinations, stupor, paralysis and even coma. The blood flow to the brain increases by 40% within 12 to 36 hours of exposure to high altitude, but falls back to normal values by the fifth day. It has been reported that a valuable addition to the treatment of cerebral oedema is the drug betamethasone.

4.4 Retinal haemorrhages

When cerebral oedema occurs in acute mountain sickness, the cerebrospinal fluid pressure rises and embarrasses venous and lymphatic return, commonly causing engorgement of the retinal veins and leading to retinal haemorrhages. After only two hours at 5330 m, retinal arteries and veins increase in diameter by about a fifth and blood flow through them increases by some 90%, with speeding up of circulation time and an increase in the retinal blood volume. The first report of the occurrence of retinal haemorrhages appeared in 1968 on workers at 5330 m on Mount Logan in Yukon territory. There is no evidence that significant alterations in intra-ocular pressure occur at high altitude to be responsible for the retinal haemorrhages. Retinal rods are very sensitive to hypoxia so that night blindness is a complication of diminished barometric pressure, as became apparent in fighter pilots during the Battle of Britain in the Second World War. Light sensitivity is impaired at elevations as low as 1520 m. A recent report suggests that both auditory sensitivity and vestibular function are weakened at high altitude.

4.5 Chronic mountain sickness

A small number of people living at altitudes exceeding 3000 m in the Andes develop a complex set of symptoms related to the heart and circulation, the lungs, the nervous system and the blood (Fig. 4-4). This condition is characterized physiologically by progressive under-ventilation of the alveolar spaces of the lung, which exaggerates even more the severe degree of oxygen lack in the blood and the heightened red cell mass and haemoglobin level. In this chronic mountain sickness, the haemoglobin level exceeds a remarkable $23 \, g \, dl^{-1}$. There is also an exaggeration of the pulmonary hypertension which characterizes the highlander. Some authorities regard chronic moun-tain sickness merely as a feature of ageing at high altitude since there is a progressive fall in ventilation of the alveolar spaces with increasing age. As a complication of the increased red cell mass there is an increased blood volume in this condition. Chronic mountain sickness was first described by Señor Monge in 1928 and hence is sometimes termed 'Monge's disease'. It is regarded by the Peruvian school of workers in the field of High Altitude Studies as an example of loss of acclimatization. It has an interesting geographical pathology in that it is confined to the Andes; this is because communities in this

40 §4.6

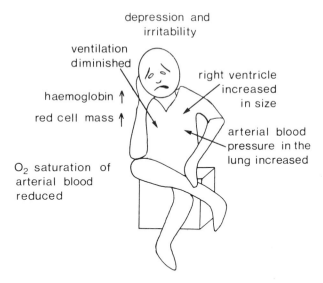

ventilation
diminished

depression and
irritability

haemoglobin ↑

red cell mass ↑

O₂ saturation of
arterial blood
reduced

right ventricle
increased
in size

arterial blood
pressure in the
lung increased

Fig. 4-4   Some of the symptoms and features of chronic mountain sickness.

area of South America exist at much higher altitude than in such
regions as the Himalayas, and because Sherpas do not produce the
high levels of haemoglobin which characterize the natural acclimatization of the Quechua (see §6.6). The simple and effective treatment of
chronic mountain sickness is to remove the affected person to live at a
lower altitude.

4.6 Abnormal haemoglobins

Haemoglobin has an important rôle in acclimatization (see §2.5).
Some variants of haemoglobin are advantageous to life at high
altitude, whereas others can prove lethal (Fig. 4-5).
HbS. This is an abnormal haemoglobin which is the basis for the
hereditary *sickle cell anaemia* in which the red cells assume a sickle
shape when exposed to a low oxygen tension. In HbS the β
polypeptide chain differs from normal adult HbA in that valine
replaces glutamic acid in the repeating amino acid groups. This
substitution causes stacking of the molecules with resulting rigid
deformity of the red cells which in turn leads to occlusion of arteries,
especially the splenic artery and its branches. This kills small portions
of the spleen cut off from their blood supply and they are converted
subsequently into scars. The extent of the tendency to sickling
depends upon the amount of HbS in the red cell as well as on the
severity of hypoxia. The genetic defect leading to the abnormal
haemoglobin and erythrocytes is virtually confined to Negroes who

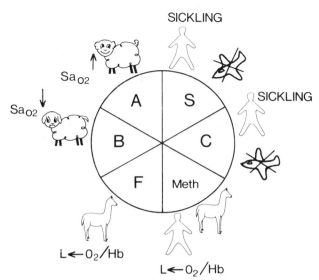

Fig. 4-5 Diagram to illustrate the significance of abnormal haemoglobins at high altitude. HbA: in sheep, maintains a high systemic arterial O_2 saturation thus favouring acclimatization to high altitude. HbB: in sheep, does not maintain high Sa_{O_2} and thus unfavourable for acclimatization. HbF: in llamas, maintains a high Sa_{O_2} and aids adaptation. HbS and HbC: in man, lead to sickling in hypoxia and make air-travel undesirable. Meth Hb: in man and llamas, interferes with uptake of O_2 by altered haemoglobin. The methaemoglobinaemia is not due to the presence of abnormal HbM.

are not, therefore, suited for life at high altitude on account of sickling and the effects on the spleen. It has become apparent that they are at risk even at the reduced cabin pressure of modern pressurized aircraft. *HbC.* HbC also predisposes air travellers and visitors to mountainous areas to the same medical consequences. It has emerged that about a quarter of persons developing infarction of the spleen on exposure to the reduced cabin pressure in aircraft have the combined sickle cell-HbC disease.

Methaemoglobin. When the ferrous iron of normal haemoglobin is converted into the ferric form, methaemoglobin is formed. This cannot combine with O_2 and, as a result, the saturation of blood with O_2 falls – methaemoglobinaemia. In view of these considerations, it is surprising that methaemoglobin has been reported as being increased at high altitude both in highlanders and indigenous animals such as the llama. Its presence in these species above 3500 m does not appear to be due to ingested chemicals or drugs. There is no evidence either that it is brought about by the appearance of the abnormal haemoglobin HbM which has a low affinity for O_2. Methaemoglobin disappears from the blood when the subject or animal descends to low altitude. Its level appears to be inversely related to the red cell count so that it is much increased in relatively anaemic subjects. It has been speculated that small amounts of methaemoglobin promote a shift of the (O_2–Hb) curve to the left providing some regulation to maintain an adequate saturation of haemoglobin with O_2 at extreme altitude, as described above.

HbF. There is a persistence of foetal type haemoglobin, HbF, in 55% of adult alpacas (*Lama pacos*) in comparison with 0.7% of adult native highlanders. This persistence of HbF with its increased affinity for O_2 shifts the (O_2–Hb) curve to the left with all its attendant advantages at high altitude.

4.7 Infection

The concentration of bacteria in ambient air decreases with altitude. Direct exposure to the increased levels of solar radiation at high altitude inhibits the growth of bacterial colonies. Studies from the Himalayas suggest higher levels of the immunoglobulin IgG are produced on arrival at high altitude and this is consistent with increased anti-viral activity and the lower reported incidence of viral disease in mountainous areas. The levels of the immunoglobulin IgM are not nearly so raised in proportion, although recent reports from India indicate that the incidence of bacterial infection is also reduced in soldiers stationed at high altitude. The levels of the immuno-globulin IgA are also raised at high altitude. Since this is dominantly present in secretions such as saliva, tears and the mucous secretions of lung and intestine, it is likely that increased IgA may assume a protective rôle at mucous surfaces at high altitude. The microbial flora of man does not appear to be influenced by the mountain environment.

Certain infections are highly characteristic of the Andean range. One is infection by *Bartonella bacilliformis* which causes Oroya fever. In this condition the organism parasitizes the red blood cells leading to a rapidly progressive anaemia with fever which may be fatal. Another manifestation of such infection is verruga peruana in which cherry-red nodules filled with the organism develop in the skin. A viral disease of high altitude is Bolivian haemorrhagic fever which is caused by the Machupo virus, one of the arenaviruses, so called because on electron microscopy the viral particles contain structures which have a fanciful resemblance to sand grains. This virus finds an animal reservoir in the wild rodent *Calomys callosus*.

4.8 Acute exposure to cold

A distinction must be made between short-term adjustment to extreme cold, in such activities as climbing, and long-term acclimatization to the low temperature innate in continuous residence in mountains. The body loses heat by convection, radiation and conduction, and by evaporation of sweat or other fluids. Each method of acute heat loss can be counteracted by suitable precautions by the climber such as avoidance of getting wet. On acute exposure to cold, skin temperature falls and the cutaneous blood flow is reduced. Hairs become erect, increasing insulation. Cold-sensitive receptors in the skin stimulate the thermostatic centre in the hypothalamus which causes the motor centres to increase skeletal muscle tone and induce shivering which may increase heat production three-fold. Shivering at high altitude is characteristic of the non-acclimatized.

4.8.1 Non-shivering thermogenesis

In contrast, there is experimental evidence to suggest that natural acclimatization to high altitude is associated with a decrease in shivering. Because man usually meets his climatic problems by avoiding them, long-term acclimatization to cold is less important than one might think. It is largely metabolic in nature and does not occur in mountaineers and newcomers ot high altitude. It is not capable of rapid utilization by the non-acclimatized. The increase in metabolism is due to non-shivering thermogenesis. It is now well established that human infants and certain newborn and adult mammals, at sea level and especially at high altitude, can increase heat production without shivering. The primary tissue responsible for non-shivering thermogenesis appears to be brown fat deposited in the abdomen, and in the cervical, interscapular, and axillary regions. The increase in metabolic rate which normally occurs after eating is reduced on exposure to high altitude. Rats already metabolically acclimatized to cold are said to be less tolerant to the hypoxia of high altitude than rats not so cold-acclimatized. It is possible that increased heat production capacity in these animals is brought about by non-shivering thermogenesis. The increase in the metabolic rate that this brings about enhances the severity of the hypoxia. There is a local vascular as well as a generalized component of acclimatization to cold in the native highlander; this takes the form of a maintenance of a high level of blood flow to the limbs such as occurs also in the Eskimo.

4.8.2 Exposure to extreme cold

Exposure to extreme cold brings about pathological conditions most unlikely to be met in long-term residents at high altitude. They will be found far more commonly in high-altitude climbers, and in air crew under war-time conditions in which there may be sudden exposure to extreme cold. Under dry freezing conditions *frostbite* may ensue. In this condition the tissues freeze with the formation of intracellular or extracellular ice crystals. A shell of skin and underlying tissue of variable depth is frozen. Plasma escapes from underlying blood vessels to form blisters. Sludging of erythrocytes occurs with the blood vessels and, together with associated constriction of the arterioles, leads to a diminution in the blood supply to the skin and subcutaneous tissues. Arteriovenous shunts appear to come into operation so that the supercooled blood from the affected area is unable to enter the general circulation. Such mechanisms increase the chance of survival but the frozen shell of tissue dies to form a 'carapace' thought to have a fanciful resemblance to the shell of a tortoise. A lesser degree of this condition is *frostnip* when supercooling of the skin leads to blanching, numbness and tingling of the extremities.

Hypothermia is a fall in body temperature which is said to begin when the level falls below 35°C and becomes lethal when the temperature of the vital organs falls to about 25°C. There is impairment of cerebration leading to delirium and confusion. There are also serious effects on the heart. Under the influence of extreme cold it may slow until there is failure of the pace-maker, i.e. specialized tissue which monitors the electrical activity and normal rhythm of the heart. There may be disturbances of the rhythm of the heart's action which range in seriousness from occasional premature beats to a total disorder of the mechanism of contraction so that the heart muscle writhes ineffectively like a bag of worms. This gross disturbance of electrical conduction within the heart and the resultant muscular contraction is termed ventricular fibrillation. Cardiac arrest may occur. Many of these effects on the heart may be related to supercooling of haemoglobin which releases O_2 far less easily. When this effect is added to those of the diminished coronary blood flow at high altitude, it is clear that the supply of O_2 to the cardiac muscle under the influence of extreme cold is barely sufficient for its needs even at rest.

4.9 Disturbances at extreme altitude

There is a critical altitude above which successful, permanent acclimatization cannot take place, and this limit appears to be somewhere around an elevation of 5500 m. Native highlanders of the Peruvian mining community of Auconquilcha in the Andes live permanently and sleep at an altitude of 5330 m, but they climb every day to their work at 5790 m refusing to sleep at this elevation. On this basis 5800 m may be defined as '*extreme altitude*'. Man can survive at elevations considerably greater than this for shorter periods but he shows features of what is termed 'high altitude deterioration'. There is an exaggeration of signs and symptoms which may be encountered at much lower elevations. Progressive muscular fatigue and mental impairment develop so that climbers may embark on foolhardy procedures or have hallucinations.

Exercise. Vigorous exercise at extreme altitude cannot be sustained above the elevation at which the maximum uptake of O_2 by the body is less than that required by the contracting muscles. The quantity of O_2 consumed by the tissues of the body *at rest* each minute is 220 to 260 ml and this demand is easily met at high altitude. On exercise, however, body requirements of O_2 may increase ten-fold to 2.6 1 min^{-1}. At sea level, the maximum oxygen uptake is 3.5 to 4.0 1 min^{-1}, but at 5800 m this capacity falls to 2.0 to 2.5 1 min^{-1}, and at 7460 m 1.3 to 1.5 1 min^{-1}. Hence, ascent into extreme altitudes causes breathing on exercise to become progressively more difficult. At a critical altitude, ventilation becomes inadequate to sustain continuous muscular exercise so that climbing becomes increasingly intermittent with the O_2 debt being repaid during periods of rest.

Lactic acid production. Acute exposure to the hypoxia of high altitude does not diminish the formation of lactic acid during severe exercise so that blood lactate levels are increased. On the other hand, chronic exposure to hypoxia reduces the amount of lactate formed. The greater the altitude, the smaller the increase in blood lactate after exhausting exercise, and the greater its rate of disappearance. This has been taken by some to be a feature of acclimatization since the buffer base at high altitude is reduced and a decreased lactate level would embarrass less such a diminished level of bicarbonate.

Thrombosis. At extreme altitude the low humidity leads to serious problems of dehydration. At 5800 m there is an appreciable loss of water through the deep, rapid ventilation. As a result, the water turnover increases from 2.9 to 3.9 1 day^{-1}. Heavy physical activity increases the turnover to 5 1 day^{-1}. Survival at extreme altitude demands on a large water intake and dehydration may be a factor in inducing serious episodes of thrombosis in young climbers. Even Sherpas have been involved in such serious catastrophes as cerebral thrombosis.

The lung in acute decompression. When the lungs of rats are exposed suddenly to a barometric pressure approaching that at the summit of Mount Everest, there are pronounced ultrastructural changes. There is swelling and destruction of the two main types of cells lining the alveolar spaces of the lung, the granular and membranous pneumocytes, with exposure of the denuded fused basement membrane of the alveolar-capillary wall. At the same time there is what almost amounts to a suction effect on the pulmonary capillaries, so that red blood cells are sucked from the capillaries into the interstitial tissue of the lung.

5 Animal Species at High Altitude

Many animal species like man have to acclimatize to survive at high altitude. Examples of species which live in mountain areas, form an extension of a common stock largely native to the surrounding lowlands, and show an increased haemoglobin level in response to the hypoxic environment, are the Russian wood mouse (*Apodemus*) and the deer mouse of White Mountain (*Peromyscus*).

5.1 Cattle

Cattle do not acclimatize well to high altitude since they have a naturally muscular pulmonary vasculature which renders them very susceptible to the development of pulmonary hypertension. Calves grazing on the highlands around Salt Lake City may develop such a degree of raised pressure in the pulmonary circulation as to die of congestive heart failure. Since this condition leads to oedema of the region between the forelegs and the neck, the 'brisket', the condition is commonly referred to as 'brisket disease'. The disease occurs only in the European type of cattle (*Bos tauros*), usually of the Ayrshire, Shorthorn, Jersey and Swiss breeds. Brisket disease is thus a *cardiopulmonary* form of loss of acclimatization based on the constrictive effect of hypoxia on the pulmonary arterioles. It is *not* a *respiratory* form of loss of acclimatization such as chronic mountain sickness which occurs in man and which is based on underventilation of the alveolar spaces in the lung (Fig. 5-1).

5.2 High-altitude camelids

In contrast to cattle, the high-altitude camelids such as the llama (*Lama glama*), the alpaca (*Lama pacos*), the guanaco (*Lama guanicoe*), and the vicuña (*Lama vicugna*), are indigenous to high altitude. Their pulmonary arteries are thin-walled and do not respond to hypoxia by constriction. This means that the llama does not increase resistance to the flow of blood through its lungs and so does not develop an increase in muscle bulk or failure of the right ventricle of the heart, as occurs in patients with lung disease predisposing to hypoxia. The carotid bodies of these animals do not appear to enlarge in response to hypoxia.

The llama (or alpaca) does not deepen its ventilation on exposure to the hypoxia of high altitude. It maintains a high arterial O_2 saturation by a higher affinity of its haemoglobin for O_2. There is a

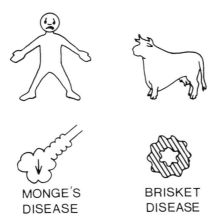

MONGE'S   BRISKET
DISEASE   DISEASE

Fig. 5-1 Diagram to illustrate the essential difference between loss of acclimatization in man and cattle. In man, the condition is chronic mountain sickness (Monge's disease) and is the result of chronic under-ventilation of the alveolar space of the lung. In cattle, the condition is brisket disease and is the result of sustained constriction of the muscularized terminal portion of the pulmonary arterial tree. Thus, the human form of loss of acclimatization is *respiratory* in nature while the bovine form is *cardiopulmonary*.

leftward shift of the (O_2-Hb) curve which is explained by a weak reaction between the haemoglobin molecule and organic phosphates in the red blood cell (Fig. 5-3). Llamas and vicuñas born and bred at high altitudes do not show high levels of haemoglobin or red cell mass as in man: diminished O_2 gradients of acclimatization are less important than increased tissue O_2 extractions of adaptation. Availability of O_2 for the tissues of camelids is also enhanced by the small, numerous red blood cells which have an ellipsiodal shape offering an increased surface area for O_2 diffusion. Thus, the very efficient utilization of O_2 by the tissues, and the ability to operate at a systemic venous O_2 pressure lower than most other species, are characteristic of animals indigenous to high altitude. Alpaca muscle also has a high myoglobin concentration.

5.3 High-altitude geese

Therefore, the *adaptation* as contrasted to *acclimatization* of high altitude camelids is associated with a weak interaction of organic phosphates and haemoglobin within red cells. There are high-altitude geese which adapt to extreme elevation in a very similar manner; for example, the bar-headed goose (*Anser indicus*) is capable of migrating across the Himalayas from India to Tibet at an altitude of 10 000 m where the ambient PO_2 is some 50 mm Hg. Another high-altitude species is the Bolivian goose (*Chlöephaga melanoptera*). Such species of goose also show a leftward shift of the (O_2–Hb) curve due to reduced interaction of 2, 3 DPG, adenosine triphosphate (ATP), or inositol pentaphosphate (IPP) and haemoglobin. In the Canada goose (*Branta canadensis*) and the greylag goose (*Anser anser*) this weak interaction does not occur.

5.4 Sheep

In the case of sheep in mountainous areas the high affinity of blood for oxygen appears to be rather an expression of the intrinsic characteristics of the type of haemoglobin present (Fig. 5-2). It is now established that the blood of healthy adult sheep contains two types of haemoglobin, A and B, which are inherited as Mendelian traits and are present in about equal amounts in the blood in heterozygotes. At high altitude, sheep carrying HbA have a mean systemic arterial O_2 saturation significantly higher than HbB carriers (Fig. 4-5). In contrast, HbB appears to be advantageous to sheep at low altitude for here the PO_2 is sufficient to achieve 90% arterial O_2 saturation, while at the same time this type of haemoglobin will ensure a plentiful release of O_2 to the tissues. On the other hand, at high altitude HbA affords an advantageous uptake of O_2 from the lung, although, of course, release of O_2 to the tissues is hindered.

5.5 Pigs

Another manner in which the (O_2–Hb) curve may be shifted to the left with increased affinity of haemoglobin for O_2 and adaptation to the hypoxia of high altitude may be due to an abnormally low concentration of relevant organic phosphates within the red cells. This occurs in foetal as contrasted to adult pigs (Fig. 5-2).

5.6 Amphibia

Telmatobius culeus is an aquatic frog of Lake Titicaca situated at an altitude of 3810 m. It is adapted to the low PO_2 in the water and to the coldness of its aquatic environment by means of a variety of developments in its morphology, physiology and behaviour. The surface area of the skin is increased by pronounced numerous large folds which hang from the back, sides and hind legs. These folds have a rich blood supply in a dense network of capillaries. The volume of the red cells is small and the red cell count high. It is clear that the specialized skin serves as a gill allowing the animal to obtain sufficient O_2 to meet its metabolic requirements. The high O_2 affinity of the haemoglobin enhances the uptake of what O_2 is available and the high red cell mass and count facilitate its transport. Furthermore,

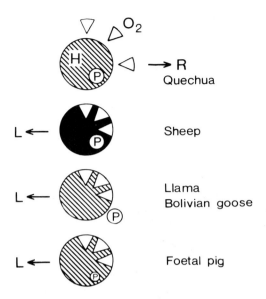

Fig. 5-2 This diagram illustrates how events within the red cell alter the affinity of haemoglobin for O_2, thus determining the shift of the (O_2–Hb) curve and the impact of this on the processes of acclimatization and adaptation as described in the text. In the **Quechua**, intraerythrocytic organic phosphates (P) such as 2, 3 DPG maintain the haemoglobin (H) in its deoxy form, thus diminishing the affinity of haemoglobin for O_2 (represented by triangles), elevating the PO_2 in the plasma, shifting the (O_2–Hb) curve to the right (**R**), and aiding acclimatization. Some **sheep** possess a type of haemoglobin, HbA which inherently has an increased affinity for O_2 thus shifting the (O_2–Hb) curve to the left (**L**). Animals indigenous to high altitude such as the **llama** and **Bolivian goose** show a weak interaction between haemoglobin and intraerythrocytic phosphates thus maintaining a high affinity of haemoglobin for O_2 which shifts the (O_2–Hb) curve to the left and aids adaptation. In the **foetal pig** there appear to be unusually low concentrations of intraerythrocytic organic phosphates which aid a high affinity of haemoglobin for O_2, and a leftward shift of the (O_2–Hb) curve.

there is the possibility that gas exchange is enhanced by increased contact between the skin and water, engineered by the frog bobbing up and down rapidly, the so called 'bobbing behaviour'.

5.7 Chicken

The lung structure and respiratory system of birds are considerably different from those of mammals. The greatest difference is the mechanism to maintain the distended state of the lungs. In the mammalian lung this is brought about by a sub-atmospheric pressure in the pleural cavity, but in birds it is due to normal lung tissue adhesions to the rib cage, and so the pulmonary circulation is independent of changes in the intrathoracic pressures. Nevertheless, the chicken responds to high altitude by a consistent pulmonary arterial hypertension. Such data are more consistent with the view that hypoxia exerts a direct effect on the vascular smooth muscle of the terminal portions of the pulmonary arterial tree than with the concept that intrathoracic and alveolar pressure may press on and close the pulmonary blood vessels.

5.8 The Aeolian community

Although man can exist for only comparatively short periods at extreme altitudes exceeding 5800 m, it has now become clear that lower forms of animal life colonize this inhospitable environment permanently. The first suspicion that this might be so arose from observations of members of the British Everest Expedition in 1924 who reported that they had seen jumping spiders of the family *Salticidae* at elevations as high as 6710 m. Life is possible at these extraordinary heights because organic debris, seeds, and pollens are carried upwards by winds and deposited on the lee sides of rocks as high as 6100 m. Fungi grow on this deposited material and form the first stage of a food chain providing nutrition for these extreme altitude dwellers. Since their survival depends on food brought upwards to them by the wind they have been named the 'Aeolian Community' after Aeolus, the god of winds.

They are members of the orders *Thysanura* and *Collembola* and thus represent the oldest and most primitive insects. The most characteristic member of the community is the Springtail, a crawling and jumping insect of the order of *Collembola* which has a trigger-like mechanism under the body capable of throwing it a few inches into the air. *Anthymiid* flies are also found, and they are eaten by the *Salticid* jumping spiders observed by the British climbers in 1924. Herbivorous and predaceous mites and small centipedes may also range above 6000 m.

6 Acclimatization and Adaptation

Men and animals living in mountain areas are not of equal biological status with regard to the high-altitude environment. The mammal may adjust to chronic oxygen deprivation in several ways (Figs 6-1 and 6-2).

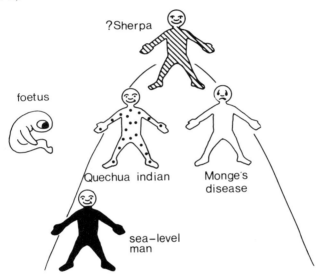

Fig. 6-1 Diagrammatic representation of the different varieties of biological status of various groups of men at high altitude. Sea-level man is indicated by the filled figure. He may undergo acquired acclimatization to emulate the natural acclimatization of the Quechua Indian of the Peruvian Andes, indicated by the stippled figure. The open figure indicates Monge's disease which is regarded by some as a respiratory form of loss of acclimatization to high altitude. Cross-hatching indicates the possibility of adaptation, as contrasted to acclimatization, in the Sherpa. The normal human foetus, at sea level or at high altitude, may be regarded as 'a little highlander' acclimatized to high altitude.

6.1 Accommodation

This term describes the initial response of man to acute exposure to hypoxia and includes such phenomena as increased ventilation and heart rate. Symptoms of accommodation are due entirely to acute hypoxia and are reversed immediately on the administration of oxygen.

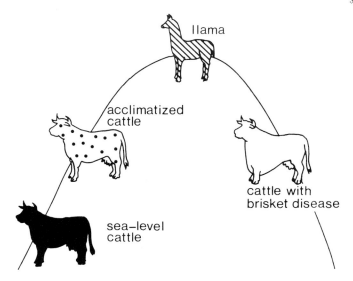

Fig. 6-2 Diagrammatic representation of the different varieties of biological status of various groups of animal at high altitude. Sea-level cattle are indicated by the filled figure. They may undergo acclimatization as indicated by the stippled figure. The open figure indicates cattle in the region of Salt Lake City affected by brisket disease which is a cardiopulmonary form of loss of acclimatization to high altitude. Cross-hatching indicates adaptation as exemplified by the llama and as described in the text.

6.2 Acquired acclimatization

This is the process by which lowlanders ascending to high altitude adjust to the hypoxia. The numerous components of acquired acclimatization were described when the transport of oxygen from air to tissues was considered (see Chapter 2).

6.3 Natural acclimatization

This is the term used to describe the processes of acclimatization found in native highlanders. It is *qualitatively* identical to acquired acclimatization but is more complete *quantitatively*. In particular, the highlander has a far greater capacity for much harder physical activity and work at high altitude than the lowlander undergoing acclimatization.

6.3.1 The native highlander

In the two major regions of the world where large communities exist at high altitudes, the Andes and the Himalayas, the native population is of Mongoloid stock (Fig. 6-3). It is likely that the physique of these native highlanders is largely determined genetically by their ethnic origin so that caution must be applied before ascribing too readily physiological advantages to their physical attributes. At the same time, it is reasonable to accept that these peoples may have undergone some anatomical or biochemical adjustments to the

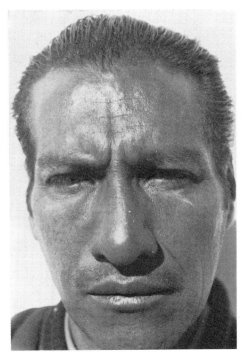

Fig. 6-3   Facial appearance of a Quechua from the Peruvian Andes living at Cerro de Pasco, a mining town situated at 4330 m. The suffused appearance of the face due to high levels of haemoglobin is striking; this is a feature of acclimatization to high altitude.

extreme environment in which they have lived for many thousands of years. One example is the barrel-shaped chest which is thought to bring beneficial effects on respiration. Certainly the 'vital capacity' is increased from childhood in the Quechuas and Aymaras. There is experimental evidence to indicate that the structure of the growing lung in the rat is influenced by the PO_2 in the atmosphere, hypoxia increasing lung volume and hyperoxia (excess of oxygen) diminishing it. However, no detailed studies of the lung by tissue morphometry have been carried out to confirm that the internal surface area of the lung of the highlander is increased compared to that of the lowlander.

The Quechuas show a remarkable predominance of blood group O. This is, however, not a feature of the highlander *per se* since in Nepal only a third of the population has this group. It is of interest that Peruvian mummies show blood groups A, B and AB and these findings are not artefactual due to bacterial contamination of the mummified tissues. It seems likely that group B has been eliminated from the Andes by natural selection.

Quechuas resemble Asiatic mongols with almond-shaped eyes with thick epicanthic folds at either side of the root of the nose (Fig. 6-3). There is a russet-red colouration of the mucous membranes due to the increased red cell mass and there is a superimposed bluish colour known as cyanosis due to the presence of more than $5\,\mathrm{g}\,\mathrm{dl}^{-1}$ of deoxyhaemoglobin brought into existence by the diminished oxygen saturation of the arterial blood. There is a curvature of the finger nails known as beaking. These native highlanders are shorter and weigh less than coastal mestizos or Caucasians. Our personal view is not to accept the concept of a 'high-altitude man'. The native highlander of the Andes probably adjusts to his environment by the processes of acclimatization just like sea-level man. These processes of 'natural acclimatization' are identical to those of acquired acclimatization but differ in extent. It also has to be kept in mind that many of the features of acclimatization shown by the Quechuas of the Andes are not shown by the Sherpas of the Himalayas.

6.3.2 *Longevity in the highlander*

There is no evidence to suggest that residence at high altitude shortens life expectancy provided chronic mountain sickness does not develop. Indeed there are remote mountainous areas of the world where people are alleged to live much longer and remain more vigorous in old age than in most modern societies. Such areas include Vilcabamba in Ecuador, the land of the Hunza in the Karakorum range of Kashmir, and the Abkhazia region of the Caucasian mountains of Georgia in the U.S.S.R. Claims of longevity in such regions are difficult to confirm because of the problems of establishing unequivocally the date of birth. In such areas the daily calorie intake tends to be low and the subjects are not obese. Most endure hard physical labour from childhood onwards. The importance of genetic factors is difficult to assess. In these communities the aged still have an important rôle in the family group, a condition no longer operating in the so-called developed countries of the West. A feeling of being wanted and needed must be an incentive to survive.

6.4 Loss of acclimatization

Loss of acclimatization may be cardiovascular in nature; this form occurs in calves in high mountain ranges in Utah where it is manifested as 'brisket disease' (see §5.1). In man, loss of acclimatization is respiratory in nature and is exemplified by chronic mountain sickness, the so-called 'Monge's disease' (see §4.5).

6.5 Adaptation

Acclimatization may be regarded as a reversible, non-inheritable change in the anatomy or physiology of an organism which enables it to survive in an alien environment. In contrast, adaptation may be regarded as the development of biochemical, physiological and anatomical features which are heritable and of genetic basis enabling the species to explore the environment of high altitude to its best advantage. In mountain areas, acclimatized man and adapted indigenous high altitude animals are found living together, both successfully. In general, a shift of the (O_2–Hb) curve to the right is indicative of acclimatization whereas a shift to the left indicates adaptation.

6.6 Adaptation v. acclimatization in 'high-altitude man'

There is an increased Bohr effect in Quechua Indians and this is to be regarded as a feature of acclimatization. This change is not to be found in Sherpas who also commonly show normal sea-level values of red cell mass. Levels of 2, 3 DPG are not raised in highland Sherpas compared to sea-level subjects. These natives of the Himalayas show a pronounced shift of the (O_2–Hb) curve to the left. All of these features are more akin to adaptation than acclimatization. Hence native highlanders may be acclimatized, if Quechua, or adapted in the case of Sherpas. It is conceivable that the Sherpas having lived in their mountain home for so much longer, perhaps half a million years, are at a more advanced biological state in coping with their adverse environmental conditions.

7 Mental Reaction and the Psyche

Electroencephalographic changes. The study of the electrical activity of the brain, *electroencephalography*, reveals that this function is modified by the hypoxia of high altitude. Irregular slow waves appear in all leads, and are of greatest amplitude in the fronto-temporal regions. The 5 Hertz (Hz) activity may be preceded by an increase in the faster alpha wave activity (8–16 Hz). Variations in Pa_{CO_2} are without effect on the characteristics of the electroencephalogram in hypoxia, but influence the level of systemic arterial saturation at which the changes occur, the higher the level of Pa_{CO_2} the lower the level of sytemic arterial oxygen saturation at which the characteristic hypoxic electroencephalographic stages are detected. Such variations probably mediate changes in cerebral oxygenation through alterations in cerebral blood flow which is linearly related to Pa_{CO_2}.

Mental reaction. There is considerable literature on testing the performance of higher cerebral function at high altitude but studies of this type must be carried out with great care and the results interpreted with caution. Decision-making tends to be impaired at high altitude but such impairment appears to be readily overcome by motivation and training. Even low blood levels of alcohol diminish the time of useful consciousness of a subject when he is suddenly exposed to hypoxia.

Hallucinations. At extreme altitudes exceeding 5800 m there is an onset of significant mental impairment with serious lapses of judgement. At such heights hallucinations may occur. Commonly these take the form of a phantom companion. Several high-altitude climbers have had the disconcerting experience of offering chocolate or mint-cake to a companion who was not there. Mountaineers occasionally report having seen strange objects, and in one classic account they took the form of bird-like creatures in the sky. On one ill-fated climb of Aconcagua (6920 m) in Argentina the climbers ascended too rapidly, became grossly disorientated, and reported having seen on the summit dead mules, trees, highway equipment and a mountain patrol.

Psyche of the native highlander and high-altitude climber. It seems that the effects of the hypoxia of high altitude *per se* on the psyche of the native highlanders of Peru are minimal. They live normal mental lives on high mountains for these are their home. The introverted withdrawn character of the Quechuas is an expression of race and ethnic origin rather than hypoxic stress.

A love of mountains and a desire to scale them is not innate in man. A terror of mountains and of the monsters supposedly lurking within them persisted for centuries. With the ascent of Mont Blanc (4810 m) in 1786, the era of high climbing began. Man largely overcomes his environmental difficulties by avoiding them. Not so the high-altitude climber who deliberately exposes himself both to physical injury and to extreme conditions of cold and hypoxia that will not support life indefinitely and which may prove fatal. A recent analysis of questionnaires by psychiatrists showed high-altitude climbers to be

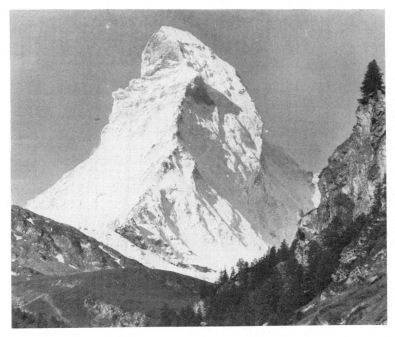

Fig. 7-1 The Matterhorn on the border between Italy and Switzerland. The dramatic conquest of this peak on July 14th 1865, marred by the controversial death of four of the party on the descent, opened an era of high-altitude climbing throughout the world.

intelligent and resourceful but aggressive, self-centred, and highly competitive! It has been suggested that for them achievement is measured in terms of thousands of feet, vertically. The very language of mountaineering is military in nature with talk of the expedition, assault, conquest and defeat. In many instances the enemy to be overcome is not only the mountain but also other competitors trying to subjugate it. This is exemplified by the story of the ascent of the

Matterhorn (Fig. 7-1) by Whymper and his party in 1865 in which rival British and Italian teams raced each other to the summit with tragic results. The conquest of the Matterhorn introduced a new unhealthy factor of nationalism to climbing which has unfortunately been reinforced by several mountaineering expeditions during this century. The new 'Man at High Altitude' is a type of sea-level man bringing with him to the mountainside his characteristics of competitive thrust and aggression so alien to the native highlander of the Andes and the Himalayas.

Mountain myths. For countless generations the Sherpas have recounted stories of the *Yeti*, a wild, hairy creature of the Himalayas. They are regarded as having several interesting physical attributes including breasts of the female that are so large they have to throw them over their shoulders when running or bending down. They are also said to be inordinately fond of alcohol. There have been numerous sightings of the Yeti in the Himalayas and many reports of big unexplained footprints in the snow which can in fact readily be explained away as body-prints of small species. Some still maintain that the Yeti is a relict form of *Gigantopithecus* but it seems more likely that the basis of the myth is the orang-utan (*Pongo pygmaeus*).

When mongoloid peoples emigrated into North America via the Bering Strait region they took the 'bigfoot' myth with them. It became known as the *Sasquatch*, an Amerindian word meaning 'the wild man of the woods'. On its introduction into the American continent the *idea* had to be transferred to a *different kind of animal*. There are no orang-utans in the New World and the selected animal was a bear.

In Europe, the mountain 'monster' took the form of a *dragon*. Until two or three centuries ago Europeans, including some members of the Royal Society, believed that the Alps were infested with such creatures. As the dragons flew through the mountains they were supposed to drop stones which had the power to effect miraculous cures of diseases such as dysentery and cholera. One of these 'dragon stones' is housed in the Museum of Natural History in Basle.

8 Practical Import of High-Altitude Studies

In their conquest of the greater peaks in the world, climbers deliberately expose themselves to the dangers of hypoxia and intense cold inherent in reaching extreme altitudes. Investigations carried out on such expeditions have deepened our understanding of man at high altitude and there is a growing realization of the practical importance of high-altitude studies. Data gained from such investigations frequently shed new light on the physiological and pathological effects of chronic hypoxia on various organs and tissues without the complications of coexisting disease to blur the lesions. A good example is the considerable impetus which has been given to investigation of the structure, function and pathological reactions of chemoreceptor tissue by studies of the carotid bodies at high altitude. Another is application of the knowledge gained on the effects of hypoxia on the pulmonary circulation from studies at high altitude to heart and lung disease.

In addition to such fundamental physiological contributions to clinical medicine, there are more direct practical applications. For example, acute mountain sickness and its more serious developments – high altitude pulmonary and cerebral oedema – are likely to prove an increasing problem in the travel industry in view of the growing popularity of trekking holidays in mountain areas such as the Himalayas. The medical profession is becoming aware of the dangers of lowlanders suddenly being transported by plane to altitudes of the order of 3660 m to begin a trekking holiday, but unfortunately, so far, this awareness does not appear to be shared by the tourist industry. In connection with the travel industry, reference has already been made (§4.6) to the dangers inherent in subjects with abnormal haemoglobins HbS and HbC ascending to high altitude or travelling in the reduced cabin-pressure of modern aircraft. Air-containing cavities in the body may expand and lead to dangerous medical emergencies in pressurized aeroplanes.

High-altitude studies also have practical relevance in times of war. The border dispute between India and China (in 1962) led to large numbers of troops being moved from sea level to high mountainous areas and an epidemic of cases of acute mountain sickness, some of which proved fatal. This campaign highlighted the need for an understanding of high-altitude problems in planning military operations in mountainous areas. Pilots of military aircraft may have to eject and suddenly expose themselves to the changes of extreme altitude. The building of high-altitude telescopes necessitates a code of practice to be followed by the staff so that acute mountain sickness or its serious complications are avoided. A current example is the new infra-red telescope built by the Science Research Council on the summit of Mauna Kea, a volcano some 4200 m high, on the island of Hawaii.

Finally, the knowledge gained on the effects of altitude on man can also be applied in a totally different field—that of athletics. The holding of the nineteenth Olympiad in 1968 in Mexico City, at an altitude of 2380 m, made it clear that the capacity of athletes to compete successfully at altitude depends not only on their individual fitness, but also on their ability to cope with the environment. At that Olympiad, Ron Clarke, from Australia, who was the world record holder in the 10 000 m event, finished sixth and in a state of collapse. The first five places were filled by athletes either native to high altitude or domiciled there for a prolonged period. Children born and brought up with moderate exercise in high-altitude areas of Kenya or New Guinea have been shown to develop an increased total lung capacity and an enhanced diffusing capacity in the lung thus favouring an early potential for athletics.

Further Reading

In this account of acclimatization and adaptation we have drawn on our personal experience of four expeditions to the Andes and have supplemented this with data from many papers on high-altitude medicine and physiology. We have thought it best not to encumber the text with detailed references which might spoil for the young reader this first encounter with a fascinating area of biology. Readers wishing to have access to a detailed bibliography on high altitude studies and a more comprehensive set of illustrations are referred to our book *Man at High Altitude* (Churchill Livingstone, Edinburgh, 1977). For the young and not so young who are more specifically interested in climbing and in the protection of high-altitude climbers from the rigours of mountaineering, especially cold, we recommend *Mountain Medicine. A Clinical Study of Cold and High Altitude* by Michael Ward (Crosby, Lockwood and Staples, St. Albans, 1975). The problems of early balloonists and present-day airmen at high altitude are considered in a most interesting manner by D. H. Robinson in *The Dangerous Sky. A History of Aviation Medicine* (G. T. Foulis, Henley-on-Thames, 1973).